Crucible is published quarterly by Hymns Ancient & Modern Ltd.
Registered Charity No. 270060

This publication is in collaboration with the Church of England's
Division of Mission and Public Affairs; the William Temple Foundation.

Correspondence and articles
Correspondence and articles for submission should be sent to the
editor via Hymns Ancient and Modern, periodicals@hymnsam.co.uk
Articles should be of about 3,000 words.

Subscriptions
(for four copies): individual rate £22; institutions £40;
individual international £40; institutional international £50;
Single copies cost £7.
All prices included postage and packing. Cheques should
be made payable to Crucible, and sent to: Crucible subscriptions,
Subscription Manager, 13a Hellesdon Park Road, Norwich NR6 5DR.

Tel: 01603 785 910   Fax: 01603 624483.
crucible@hymnsam.co.uk

Direct Debit forms available from the same address

ISSN 0011-2100
ISBN 978-0-334-03162-8

H
Y
M
N
S
**Ancient
&Modern**

Contents

Editorial

Editorial

CAROL WARDMAN

In the midst of change, the world urgently needs to rediscover a moral compass: that is the common message from contributors to this edition of Crucible, examining high-profile issues with a global reach. The climate emergency, globalization, modern slavery and racism are all connected, not just as equally international problems, but in practical terms too – with elements of each feeding into and exacerbating each other.

In the day-by-day uncertainty of the summer of 2021, a whole article on overseas aid risked being out of date before the ink was dry (or the electrons had settled); but as world-wide problems demand international solidarity and cross-cutting solutions, a chunk of this introduction will glance over our fraught response to poverty and inequality on a global scale.

You might not expect the first words from a former vice squad officer of the Metropolitan Police, Head of the Met's Human Trafficking Unit and the UK's first Independent Anti-Slavery Commissioner, to be a quote from Pope Francis; but Kevin Hyland and Alison Ussery set their analysis of the state of modern slavery, in the UK and the wider world, within the context of our planetary stewardship, and of our Christian duty to care for the poor, the marginalized, the voiceless, the dispossessed.

Showing what you can do if you're the Pope, Pope Francis summoned the world's leading police chiefs and bishops to a summit at the Papal Residence in 2014. This led to the Santa Marta Declaration and the formation of the Santa Marta Group: a ground-breaking global attempt to find ways of tackling a problem that can be solved only by international co-operation and determination at the highest level, by bringing together Catholic bishops, law-enforcement agencies, lawyers, and NGOs. This isn't pasting awareness-raising posters on toilet doors (although that undeniably has its place in local campaigns); this is an expert-led international effort to tackle the detection, conviction rate and prevention of a crime which is set to outstrip the drugs trade in its global value.

Modern slavery takes many forms, occurs all over the world, and – like the climate crisis and racism – is grounded in the arrogant assumption that some human beings can treat other human beings as simply there to be exploited. Like environmental degradation and racism, it is a sin in which the rich world is implicated through the unclear provenance of the products we enjoy or rely on. There is a more direct causality between climate change and racism and modern slavery, too (as the Santa Marta Group's excellent website reminds us): famine, poverty, and loss of homeland drive desperate refugees into the clutches of traffickers who lock them into exploitative, degrading or unregulated labour, where they then become invisible amongst an army of casual or migrant workers, liable as 'illegal immigrants' to fall foul of immigration laws.

Hyland and Ussery raise another important ethical question for Christians: it is our duty not just to provide food for the hungry, shelter for the homeless, etc, but also (as mentioned in the Anglican Five Marks of Mission) to question and challenge the failing structures that prevent effective action to combat injustice. The UK's well-meaning National Referral Mechanism (NRM) is manifestly under-resourced, leaving literally thousands of victims in limbo for years even before a decision is made about whether or not there are 'conclusive grounds' for proceeding under the Modern Slavery Act. During this time victims may disappear without trace: back to their homes, countries, or even into repeated exploitation; whilst the conviction rate is too pitifully small (less than 1% of slavery crimes worldwide) to deter the criminal exploiters.

The slogan "Black Lives Matter" may have been heard before 2020, but the shockingly blatant murder of George Floyd by a police officer in Minneapolis last summer brought the lethal implications of racism, quite literally, before our very eyes. Consciences smote us on both sides of the Atlantic. And so 'taking a knee' – seen since 2016 as a sporting protest by Black players in the USA during the pre-match National Anthem – became a gesture of repentance and solidarity in Britain and Europe, amongst groups as disparate as football teams and cathedral clergy, Metropolitan police officers (even in Downing Street!), and village green demonstrators. It remains to be seen whether or not the revulsion at racism at all levels, from under-expectations of Black school students to discrimination in employment or promotion, poorer outcomes in healthcare to straightforward attacks and abuse in the street or the media, will translate into a genuine change of heart and practice.

On the subject of racism, Edward Cardale combines personal reminiscence of his student days in the hotbed of USA protest politics of the 1970s with an analysis of how Christianity – and in particular, the radical theology of Union Theological Seminary, New York – influenced the Civil Rights and similar movements, and still exerts an influence today.

We are reminded of the varying roles Christianity has played in the ensuing years: from the compassionate but short-lived presidency of Jimmy Carter, through the largely single-issue (abortion) Christian Right, now blended with vaccine scepticism and climate-change denial, to the extraordinary romance between evangelical fundamentalists and Donald Trump. Cardale leaves us with definite signs of hope, now surprisingly focused in the person of Joe Biden. Arguably still the most powerful of world leaders, Biden faces criticism, perhaps even ostracism, from his church, for his principled stand against imposing his religious opinions on others through government policy (the abortion thing again); but his genial demeanour belies a surprisingly steely approach to world affairs, and Cardale wonders if under him, American religion can even now be part of the solution, rather than adding to the problem.

Stuart Elliott takes up the theme of climate-change denial, including from a Christian perspective, in his challenging piece on the urgency of environmental action. Asked to write something about COP26, and the most global issue in the world today, Elliott bucked the temptation merely to encourage world leaders and applaud the efforts of campaigners. He refuses to be dazzled by the glamour of an international summit and lays starkly before us the kind of measures we need to take, both governmentally and personally, to avoid climatic disaster on an utterly irreversible scale.

Like an addict realizing the need to change only after recognizing that they have hit rock bottom, we need to see that our 'glass is empty' (not half-full of wishful optimism or feeble hope in technology), before we shall be able to turn around our current disastrous trajectory. There is a link between global capitalism and climate breakdown, and Elliott introduces us to some startlingly original readings of scripture to jolt us into a new understanding of our place in the world and the role of the economy, alongside real-life examples of alternative approaches which show that another way is possible. The urgency of success in Glasgow this November cannot be overstated.

Stephen Green examines the 'dialogue' between the traditional Western and the Chinese world-views. Like Cardale on the USA and Elliott on the climate crisis, he sees the world-as-we-know-it on the cusp of a profound change. The turnover here is a move away from the belief that the Western, democratic, ambitious, individualistic approach – tempered (at least in modern times) by an understanding of human rights and ideals of fairness and equality within the rule of law – is the one and only, universal and best outcome for human flourishing. In its place comes a recognition that other views of the individual and society may be equally valid and beneficial. Although alternative world-views do appear from time to time in modern Western societies – think of experiments in community or communal living (not forgetting religious communities), self-sufficiency and alternative or circular economics – Green argues that in China we see a vast, industrialised and commercially successful country based on the world-view of Confucianism. This world-view is communitarian rather than individualistic, has a sense of the human place in the cosmos rather than a belief in human 'exceptionalism' (to borrow the term often used for American self-understanding!), and sees relationships between people on a group level imposing a sense of duty and obligation ahead of personal rights.

There is fascinating comparison between Chinese and Western (Greek, Jewish, Christian) philosophy, and in case we start to feel out of our depth, Green encouragingly says that neither is more Christian than the other. He finds a common understanding of the creative tension between mercy and righteousness, justice and benevolence, charity and equity – however the core qualities are described – across all traditions.

If all that sounds like a rosy view in light of the Chinese government's behaviour towards the Uighurs, independent Christians, or citizens of Hong Kong – not to mention the colossal contribution to carbon output of China's developing cities and consumer culture – Green points out that the Western world-view is equally flawed and badly implemented, and both sides would do well to 'look in the mirror of their own principles' to put things right.

Global problems demand the solution of concerted global action; and in the face of all this, the UK Government has reneged on its commitment to spend 7p in every £10 of Gross National Income on overseas aid.

The face and purpose of 'overseas aid' (perhaps more correctly, 'overseas development aid', ODA) has mutated repeatedly. Colonial powers in the early 20th century used it to provide infrastructure and facilitate the exploitation of raw materials to help their colonies emulate and support their own economic development, whilst the support of rich and powerful nations – from expansionist 19th Europeans to Cold War rivals, to China and America in the present day – subtly or blatantly encourages ideological, trading and military support from emerging players. As we come to recognise our inter-connectedness as not just fellow-members of the human race, but as co-tenants of our planetary home, equally vulnerable to emergencies from climate change to pandemics, the notion of 'global solidarity' has come to replace the 'aid' word. Global learning becomes less of a one-way system, and more of a mutual enterprise.

Before state aid became a thing, Christian missionaries added value to their evangelism with educational and humanitarian projects. All too often this focused on introducing Christianity and trousers to the unsuspecting locals; but Christian missionaries and those they inspired have also championed indigenous rights and promoted nation-building – from the Jesuits in Latin America (heroically depicted in the film *The Mission*) to the Community of the Resurrection's Anglican Mission in South Africa (nurturing Bishop Trevor Huddleston, schoolboy Desmond Tutu, and the anti-apartheid movement). Another example would be current climate change resilience led by the Methodist Church on islands in the Pacific.[1] Aiming to make the

---

[1] https://www.methodist.org.uk/media/5862/wcr-julia-edwards-mar-apr2013.pdf accessed 22.07.2

7

Crucible October 2021

Bible available in the vernacular, missionaries studied and translated indigenous languages, generating the unintended consequence of preserving them against eradication by cultural imperialists.

Medical treatment and care have benefitted from missionary work, carried out with sometimes self-sacrificing solidarity. Explorer and linguist Mary Moffat Livingstone (David was often introduced as her husband[2]) was one of many to succumb to malaria in Africa, whilst her contemporary and compatriot Mary Slessor is perhaps the best-known for early work amongst malaria sufferers. Missionaries pioneered vaccination programmes and risked early versions of the jabs on themselves. Fr (now Saint) Joseph Damien, ministering to the Hawaiian leper colony of Molokai in 1884, addressed his flock with the famous words "My fellow lepers", after contracting the disease himself. Christianity's record on HIV/AIDS has been mixed, but at least some missionary work has been directed towards overcoming stigma and teaching realistic health and safety practices.

It was a coalition of Christian humanitarian and development agencies which led to the founding, in 1992, of the UK Fairtrade Foundation, followed in 1997 by Fairtrade International. Through linking producers, importers, retailers, consumers and community groups across the world, the Fairtrade mark promotes ethical business development and equitable trading relationships as a sustainable way out of poverty. The Fairtrade scheme isn't perfect: some operations fall into the same elitist traps as conventional business, with perks of executive dining-rooms and toilets for senior staff; community facilities like schools and clinics may be free of charge only to partners in the Fairtrade scheme, not to the wider population; producers may find accreditation off-puttingly expensive, and inspection regimes may be superficial due to the costs involved. Even Fairtrade cannot create immunity to endemic food insecurity, but it can and does improve productivity, provide a decent return, facilitate access to education, and combat labour exploitation.[3] (And after all, who can argue with good works based on coffee and chocolate?)

It was Christian agencies, too, which spear-headed the millennium's

[2] https://www.wikiwand.com/en/Mary_Moffat_Livingstone accessed 22.07.21
[3] https://www.sciencedirect.com/science/article/pii/S2211912421000456 accessed 22.07.21

Jubilee 2000 campaign – "the high-water mark of international aid" as one speaker to the Christian Aid AGM in 2017 described it. This was to cancel or reduce the crippling debts of poor countries suffering from 'structural adjustment', ie the cancellation of state investment in essential services which the rich world takes for granted, like health and education, after the oil and financial crises of the 1970s.

The figure of 0.7% of GNI, as an allocation to ODA by rich countries, was first mooted by Robert McNamara, Head of the World Bank from 1968-81. Britain adopted it as a pipe-dream under the Labour Government of 1979; but in 2014 Britain led the EU in achieving and enshrining it in law, under the Conservative premiership of David Cameron.

Seven years and one pandemic later, Boris Johnson's government has scrapped it, on the grounds that the means-related figure was no longer affordable against the demands of rebuilding the economy. Despite vigorous campaigning by charities, churches, opposition and rebel MPs, it has so far proved impossible to overturn the decision, with the latest attempt resulting in conditions for its restoration which have only been met twice in the past 20 years. And despite assurances that women and girls would remain a priority, figures from the (newly re-merged) Foreign, Commonwealth and Development Office reveal that girls' education comes ninth out of the ten spending categories listed.[4] (In a gloriously easy sum to work out, from the figures given, this amounts to £10 per pupil, for the 40 million girls they aim to support across 25 countries.)

Inequality, the climate crisis, refugee displacement, racism and unrest will not be improved by cutting support to the poorest, reducing expenditure on health and education worldwide, and putting at risk the infrastructure and co-operation to combat international organised crime. There can be no better example of the urgent need to re-set the moral compass.

The Revd Canon Carol Wardman is based in Cardiff. She is the Bishops' Adviser for Church and Society, for the Church in Wales.

4 https://www.gov.uk/government/speeches/uk-official-development-assistance-oda-allocations-2021-to-2022-written-ministerial-statement accessed 25.06.21

— Modern Slavery & — Human Trafficking

KEVIN HYLAND AND ALISON USSERY

Pope Francis has called modern slavery "A scourge that wounds the dignity of our weakest brothers and sisters," and describes our contemporary world as "marked by a utilitarian perspective that views others according to the criteria of convenience and personal gain."[1]

These words sadly reflect the truth of the current stewardship of this planet, and without radical change the legacy we leave behind for generations to come might be one of divided communities: those with wealth and privilege, and those who are marginalised and seen as weak or even disposable.

Legal and factual background

The human trafficking agenda has been a subject of international debate for more than 20 years. In 2000 the United Nations agreed the Protocol to Prevent, Suppress and Punish Trafficking in Persons, Especially Women and Children (Palermo Protocol)[2]. The USA introduced the Trafficked Victims Protection Act Public Law (No: 115-393)[3], which brought about the establishment of the Department of State's Office to Monitor and Combat Trafficking in Persons along with the appointment of the US Trafficking in Persons Ambassador. This office annually publishes the TIP Report, which grades national responses in the actions taken against human trafficking, identifying countries performing significantly below expectations, which then face potential sanctions for inadequate efforts.

In 2005 the Council of Europe introduced its own Convention,[4] setting

---

[1] https://www.vaticannews.va/en/pope/news/2020-08/pope-francis-human-trafficking-scourge-against-dignity.html
[2] https://www.ohchr.org/en/professionalinterest/pages/protocoltraffickinginpersons.aspx
[3] https://www.congress.gov/115/plaws/publ393/PLAW-115publ393.pdf
[4] https://ec.europa.eu/anti-trafficking/legislation-and-case-law-international-legislation-council-europe/council-europe-convention-action_en#:~:text=The%20Convention%20of%20the%20Council,prosecuting%20those%20responsible%20for%20it.

out the framework and legislation European nations should adopt to combat human trafficking. The Convention includes guidance on the role of governments, law enforcement, border agencies, children's services, prosecutors and non-government agencies. This Convention places great importance on protection and support for victims, the non-punishment principle and 'non-refoulement' as required in the 1951 Refugee Convention. The Council of Europe established a Group of Experts (GRETA) who conduct periodic reviews and publish reports of member states' compliance with the Convention.

In England and Wales, the first trafficking legislation was introduced in 2003 and 2004, further strengthened in 2010 by the Coroners and Justice Act. However, the legislation had deficits and loopholes, and failed to provide statutory protection for victims. In 2015 the UK Modern Slavery Act[5] received Royal Assent as the final Act of Parliament before the general election.

Later that same year the United Nations agreed the 15-year strategy of 17 Global Goals, (SDGs), including target 8.7 to eradicate modern slavery by 2030, and the worst forms of child labour and child soldiers by 2025[6].

The multilateral conventions and protocols have seen most UN nations introduce domestic legislation criminalising human trafficking, but few yet provide real support for victims. Even where they do, implementation of measures is insufficient.

The international definition of this crime states:
"Trafficking in human beings shall mean the recruitment, trans-portation, transfer, harbouring or receipt of persons, by means of the threat or use of force or other forms of coercion, of abduction, of fraud, of deception, of the abuse of power or of a position of vulnerability or of the giving or receiving of payments or benefits to achieve the consent of a person having control over another person, for the purpose of exploitation."[7] (United Nations).

---

[5] https://www.legislation.gov.uk/ukpga/2015/30/contents/enacted

[6] https://sdgs.un.org/goals

[7] https://www.ohchr.org/en/professionalinterest/pages/protocoltraffickinginpersons.aspx#:~:text=(a)%20%22Trafficking%20in%20persons,giving%20or%20receiving%20of%20payments

Crucible October 2021

"Exploitation shall include, at a minimum, the exploitation of the prostitution of others or other forms of sexual exploitation, forced labour or services, slavery or practices similar to slavery, servitude or the removal of organs,"[8] *(Article 4 Council of Europe Convention).*

The UK Modern Slavery Act is arguably one of the better examples of legislation. It creates two offences that hold a maximum penalty of life imprisonment, one for slavery, servitude and forced labour, and the other for human trafficking.

Slavery, servitude and forced or compulsory labour

Section 1(1)A person commits an offence if –
(a) the person holds another person in slavery or servitude and the circumstances are such that the person knows or ought to know that the other person is held in slavery or servitude, or

(b) the person requires another person to perform forced or compulsory labour and the circumstances are such that the person knows or ought to know that the other person is being required to perform forced or compulsory labour.

Human trafficking

Section 2(1) A person commits an offence if the person arranges or facilitates the travel of another person ("V") with a view to V being exploited.

The act introduces a statutory defence where an offence is committed as a direct consequence of being trafficked.

Defence for slavery or trafficking victims who commit an offence

Section 45(1)A person is not guilty of an offence if—
(a) the person is aged 18 or over when the person does the act which constitutes the offence,
(b) the person does that act because the person is compelled to do it,
(c) the compulsion is attributable to slavery or to relevant exploitation, and

---

[8] https://ec.europa.eu/anti-trafficking/sites/default/files/cets_197.docx.pdf

(d) a reasonable person in the same situation as the person and having the person's relevant characteristics would have no realistic alternative to doing that act.

It brought a global first legislating for transparency in business supply chains and the world's only anti-slavery commissioner, to spearhead UK national and international efforts. It allows for reparation to victims and risk and prevention orders providing opportunities for prevention by police, the National Crime Agency and Immigration Enforcement to apply to courts for control measures to be imposed on those where intelligence indicates involvement in trafficking crimes or following release from custody for a human trafficking conviction anywhere in the world. To date use of these powers remains limited.

Section 50 of the act provided great hope allowing the secretary of state to make regulations for public authorities on measures when supporting suspected victims of modern slavery.

Regulations about identifying and supporting victims
Section 50 (1) The Secretary of State may make regulations providing for assistance and support to be provided to persons—
(a) who there are reasonable grounds to believe may be victims of slavery or human trafficking;
(b) who are victims of slavery or human trafficking.
(2) The Secretary of State may make regulations providing for public authorities to determine (for the purposes of regulations under subsection (1) or other purposes specified in the regulations) whether-
(a) there are reasonable grounds to believe that a person may be a victim of slavery or human trafficking;
(b) a person is a victim of slavery or human trafficking.
(3) Regulations under subsection (2) may in particular make provision about the public authorities who may make such determinations, and the criteria and procedure for doing so.

Section 50 of the Modern Slavery Act has not actually been implemented since being enacted by the UK Parliament, and the plight of victims has significantly worsened over the last few years. This section is crucial to provide local resources and support for victims.

In ratifying the Council of Europe Convention on Human Trafficking in

2009, the UK committed to providing a National Referral Mechanism (NRM). The purpose of an NRM is to allow for proactive identification of victims, and for their recovery to be provided by the Government. However, understanding of what an NRM should provide and the implementation of the Convention's 47 Articles remains weak in the UK and in most countries. An absence of understanding of the Council of Europe Convention, particularly the NRM, is a major cause of the failings in effective response to human trafficking. This could not be more evident than in the UK with the current situation.

Over the past 6 years referals to the NRM have grown from 2,337 in 2014 to 10,613 in 2020. Of the total in 2020, 92 per cent were referred by government agencies including police, immigration and local authorities, with 8 per cent coming from the NGO sector. The increase in referrals is welcomed, but this is only an administrative audit. The true test is in the levels of support provided.

Once an individual is referred to the NRM and is given a reasonable grounds decision, the referral will be considered by the Single Competent Authority (SCA) within the Home Office before a conclusive grounds decision is made. Throughout this period of time the person is living in a state of limbo with their future plans on hold. In 2020, 8,665 (82 per cent) of referrals awaited a conclusive grounds decision, and a further 9,447 referrals were also awaiting a conclusive grounds decision from previous years, meaning that at the start of 2020 over 18,000 individuals were awaiting decisions.

In 2014, despite there only being 2,339 cases, over 47 per cent (1,118) were given conclusive status as a victim of trafficking. In 2020, referrals reached 10,613 cases with outstanding cases from previous years of at least 9,447 (total of more than 20,000), and only 17 per cent (3,454) received a conclusive decision.

Most victims in the UK must endure over 18 months for a decision to confirm their status as a victim, with some taking over 3 years. During this time many do not have the right to work or education. They find it hard or impossible to access psychological support and receive derisory amounts to live on. For example, a pregnant woman believed to be trafficked receives just an additional £5 per week, not even enough to cover travel fares to prenatal appointments.

If the resources of the State are unable to negotiate the complexities of human trafficking, how can members of society make a difference? What can individuals or a group of people of faith do? Everyday opportunities to help those in need slip by. Despite the many legal instruments and commitments outlined already, the victims of traffickers all too easily become victims of failings by the State, with some regretting ever seeking support.

People of faith and those of goodwill are in a unique position to change the current situation, not just for individual victims, which is crucial, but also at a policy level with police, local government, healthcare, employers and many others who have a role in prevention or responding to this crime.

Simplifying our response

In the Gospel of Matthew (25: 31-40), we read the Judgement of Nations, as in *"When I was hungry you gave me food, I was thirsty and you gave me drink, I was a stranger and you welcomed me."* This provides a foundation for how people of goodwill, irrespective of their religion, faith or social status, should react to the needy and marginalised in our world. If we serve the 'least of these' in our communities and our world, we are serving the Lord.

Biblical teachings are very clear that we are to care for fellow human beings and to *"love our neighbour,"* (Matthew 22). In his ministry Jesus demonstrated numerous times his compassion and care for the poor and downtrodden, as he reached out without judgement or prejudice to those in need in such practical ways.

Throughout both the Old and New Testaments the message of love and compassion is clear, as the heart of God is revealed. Persecution of the weak by the strong is offensive to God, for we are taught to *"act justly, to love mercy and to walk humbly with our God,"* (Micah 6:8).

Meetings of heads of state, business meetings of chief executives or multilateral forums often place success on agreeing a principle, or a future deal, or a commitment. St Matthew's Gospel speaks of deeds in action, not merely words.

So, what can a community, congregation or people of goodwill do?

Crucible October 2021

Perhaps the first and most important step is to understand the issue. What does it mean to be a victim of human trafficking? Exploitation can derive from various means, from a minor deception to threats, serious harm and violence. Some cases including in the UK have ended in deaths, while others have been intercepted at an early stage before exploitation occurred. Perpetrators do not care whom they exploit, so men, women, young people and children may fall prey to the deception of someone who wants to benefit by abusing them. Perpetrators find a vulnerability as a means to take control and deprive that person of their freedom and human rights.

Forms of exploitation can be vastly different. In the UK human trafficking exploitation has been found in car washes, fast food outlets, brothels, nail bars, hotels, agricultural settings, on fishing vessels, and street begging. Forced criminality includes drugs cultivation and charity collecting. These examples show the complexity of this crime. There are agreed indicators of identification of victims outlined by the International Labour Organisation[9], but there is no guidance or indicators of venues. Creating a list of indicators for local communities would be an excellent project that would require detailed local knowledge.

Human trafficking and modern slavery offences may happen anywhere in the UK, in our cities, towns and rural areas. Prevention must be a priority in reaching out to our communities, and this should be done through evidence-based action and strategies delivered to young people and school children, migrants, the homeless and others who might find themselves in vulnerable situations. Church congregations and faith communities have a significant role to play in raising awareness, teaching about the signs and indicators, and providing practical support for those at risk or actual victims of exploitation.

For people of faith, the message on this agenda is clear. We are to *"learn to do right, seek justice, defend the oppressed, take up the cause of the fatherless, and plead for the widow,"* (Isaiah1:17). In today's society this must also include the victims of modern slavery and human trafficking, and we have a responsibility to speak out, challenge systems and to act and care for all.

---

[9]https://www.ilo.org/global/topics/forced-labour/publications/WCMS_203832/lang--en/index.htm

On the wider global perspective, it is essential that there is a high level strategic buy-in with political will, based on effective monitoring by meaningful metrics. Areas of responsibility must be placed into legislation and policy, bringing accountability across sectors, corporates and individuals.

Globally we need to drive out the root causes of this tragedy, with a focus on the profit generated by human trafficking and modern slavery, not just the proceeds of crime. Currently, multilateral businesses have faced penalties of over $200 million for data breaches. Or again, a $2.8 billion fine was exacted for tampering with emission readings for cars. So there are these large sanctions for failing to maintain quality control standards and penalties for employing undocumented workers. And yet, commercial enterprises small and large all too often retain profit derived from work or services at the hands of an exploited child, woman or man.

Who makes the money? Who is exploited?
- The 15-year-old child I met in Lampedusa, raped daily in connection houses in Libya to secure her passage across the Mediterranean, expecting treasures but destined to a life of exploitation, generating enormous sums for criminals at every stage.
- The mother I met in Nigeria whose son was killed by his traffickers, the financial payment for a false promise of work not only taking family savings: this cost him his life.
- The fisherman I met in Dublin, kept on board a vessel despite being injured, receiving little or no pay and subject to racial taunts and threats.
- The British girl trafficked at the age of 14, traded as a commodity for sexual gratification by British men.
- The children in the mines excavating mica for cosmetics or pearlescent paint, or cobalt to meet increasing demand for battery-powered items. Too many children's lives being destroyed and lost.

These are the kind of activities making an estimated $150 billion per year generated by this crime.

Positive steps
The US Tariff Act has been a great driver of reform, the UK and Australian Modern Slavery Acts now bring business to the agenda

with compulsory reporting, and France has a Due Diligence of Human Rights Protection. All have made some change, but it is not enough.

Globally we need to remove the possibility of commercial profit from human trafficking by introducing a notion of 'tainted money': stripping profits to provide reparation and fund the fight. This can be a real driver for a change in moral leadership, where humans are no longer a commodity for sale and exploitation. It will require positive action – such as we have already seen in, for example, data protection, security against terrorism, and many other global governance rules – which we now accept in our daily lives.

This will take determination and great leadership, placing people in the front of the queue, particularly those who are vulnerable as a new world order emerges from the COVID 19 pandemic.

We need to see meaningful implementation of international instruments and the multilateral commitments at the UN, the G20 and in the Bali Process. The words on paper need to become actions, supported with the necessary finances and resources.

If we do not take this opportunity now, the aims of the Sustainable Development Goals may be lost for generations to come. As bad as our current predicament may be, it provides an opportunity to reflect, to lead and re-emerge. The moral compass must be set, in order to break the practice of modern slavery and human trafficking in all its forms, in the next decade.

Kevin Hyland *was the UK's first Independent Anti-Slavery Commissioner (2014-2018) and currently Ireland's representative to the Council of Europe Independent Group of Experts for Trafficking. He is chief adviser to the Santa Marta Group, chairs the Responsible Recruitment Group of the Institute of Human Rights and Business and the Island of Ireland Human Trafficking Project, and provides strategic leadership to the OSCE in producing global victim support guidance.*

Alison Ussery *has a background in community development and education in North Eastern Romania and the Balkans. She has been involved in anti-modern slavery work in Wales since 2013, and is the founder of the charitable organisation Haven of Light, which focuses on* *awareness, prevention, and advocacy for those at risk of slavery and trafficking; and she is a Board member of the European Freedom Network.*

— Christianity, race and — politics in the USA

EDWARD CARDALE

Since the civil rights era of the 1960s, the mighty USA has seen many hopes raised and dashed in its slow, faltering progress towards racial justice in its own society.

One bastion of liberal Christianity has reflected not only the wavering hopes and fortunes of this movement, but also the belief that a Christian America could re-discover its better self. The path ahead for those engaged in that struggle now looks as formidable as ever.

Introduction: background to the struggle

In 1973, with an Oxford theology degree behind me, I was preparing for ordained ministry. A year in the rural college setting of Cuddesdon, near Oxford, taught me that a quiet disciplined routine of prayer, study and formation was what I needed for my future life as a priest. But a second year at Union Theological Seminary in the City of New York showed me that ministry was about responding, immediately, to the urgent demands of a liberal Christian agenda. That year offered me less time for prayer or liturgy, and much more time for a radical engagement with the modern world.

It was both alarming and exhilarating. Within days of arriving in New York, I was meeting and eating with fellow students whose lives were a world away from the white male Anglican community I had left behind. They included a radical Catholic priest and his followers who had fronted the anti-Vietnam War movement with the Berrigan brothers, and numerous women who were blazing a trail for future ministry, sometimes in various states of conflict with their own sponsoring churches. And there were more conventional students like me, for whom Christian liberation took on new meaning as we heard from fiery academics like the young Black professor James H. Cone.

Justice and Peace were the watchwords, for countless Christian communities and activist groups. The ending of the war in Vietnam, though a vindication of sorts for the anti-war movement energised by the religious left and a much larger coalition, came to stand for a gradual decline in American authority across the world, which has continued ever since. World peace, in the sense of the avoidance of a major international war, has been maintained. But it has been partial and unconvincing, even more so in the light of all that followed 9/11.

Justice, particularly within the USA, has arguably made less progress. And the struggle for racial justice and equality in our times has been harder and more intractable, it seems, than the movements for women's rights and sexual minorities. The quest for the rights of American ethnic minorities has run into the sands of endless political and cultural division.

Slavery was abolished after the Civil War in the 1860's, but it took another century before racism, segregation and prejudice began to be outlawed or addressed more seriously. Thus, for example, the worst single (recorded) outbreak of racist hate and violence after the Civil War took place in Tulsa, Oklahoma, in 1921. It has with good reason been described as the Tulsa race massacre.

The passing of the Civil Rights Bill in 1965 marked a moment of great progress, but the zenith of American liberalism in the 1960's has neither fully matured nor recovered from the setbacks and failures of the past 50 years. The promise of racial justice, embodied in the iconic life of Martin Luther King and enshrined for ever in his 1963 '*I have a dream*' speech in Washington D.C., has not been able to bend the 'arc of history' clearly toward social and racial justice in American society.

The witness of a liberal theological institution

My aim in this article is to offer a glimpse of how Christian witness was not only the life-blood of civil rights and other movements in the past, but still has remarkable significance for the struggle that lies ahead, in this truly perilous era for American democracy and the future of its entire polity. I shall look through the 'lens' of this one institution, Union Theological Seminary in the City of New York, to observe a few sweeping trends, before looking at wider religious influences on the search for political justice.

Union Theological Seminary in the 1970's was trying to renew its academic role in the post-Vietnam period. Union was still a world-renowned centre of theological excellence. The names of the theological giants who had taught there – Niebuhr, Tillich, Bonhoeffer – were on the lips of faculty and students alike, and their legacies lived on. It was primarily 'liberal Protestant' but it could also be seen as 'ecumenical Christian'. Thus Roman Catholics such as Haring and Kung were often visiting faculty members, and the outstanding Catholic scholar Raymond E. Brown was a permanent professor of biblical studies. Union was also breaking ground with the appointment of Black and feminist scholars who were blazing a new trail for both American and worldwide churches.

But Union was also, financially and institutionally, heading for the rocks. The full story is told in a recent book celebrating the life and work of the man who was appointed President in 1975: Christian Ethics in Conversation: A Festschrift in honor of Donald W. Shriver Jr. Shriver was brought up in Virginia, and his early life as a student and a young Presbyterian minister in North Carolina was surrounded by the realities of a segregated society in which Black Americans were treated as second-class human beings. Segregation in the southern states was as much accepted by the churches as it was in the society to which they belonged. Shriver's evolution into a visionary prophetic Christian leader, inspired by the teachings of both Richard and Reinhold Niebuhr among others, is replicated in many who have begun their journey in conservative Christian homes or churches, but have responded to a more radical call of God upon their lives.

When he arrived in New York in 1975, he was faced with the unenviable task of rescuing Union from its deepening crisis. It was a crisis brought on by the decline of liberal Christianity and the loss of confidence in a prophetic and ethical role for the churches. For this task Donald Shriver was wonderfully equipped, though it was a massive undertaking to steer such an independent-minded institution away from actually hitting the rocks, and to find, eventually, a new and viable course.

Our interest here is less in his many gifts of leadership, and more in the important writings which illustrate his lifelong witness to the cause of racial justice and reconciliation. As a White southerner, Shriver knew from years of personal experience the suffering of his

Black fellow-citizens in the context of what Martin Luther King called 'the scourge of racism'. He demonstrated in the many facets of his life – spiritual, ecclesial, academic, ethical and political – what it meant to oppose that scourge. His first book of edited sermons was *The Unsilent South: Prophetic Preaching in Racial Crisis (1965)*.

Later, his greatest impact came through two books which show his honest wrestling with human flaws including racism in himself, other people, and society. He has never flinched from exploring the ethical dilemmas of seeking forgiveness (and reparation) for past evils, while not reducing commitment to practical resolution of conflicts, whether in international relations abroad or race relations at home. Cornel West sums him up by declaring, with reference to some of the well-known leading lights of Union's story, that the genius of Shriver was to wed the best of liberal evangelicalism, the unclassifiable creativity of Tillich and Niebuhr, and the emerging liberation theologies of James Cone, Beverly Harrison and others.

His legacy to Union Seminary was not merely reforming a great academic institution but also in the appointment of faculty members, and in the policies which have seen widening opportunities for Black scholars and students, going way beyond the long and remarkable career of James H. Cone.

One chapter of the Festschrift by Eric Mount is titled A Lover's Challenge to America. Here we see the characteristic combined love and exasperation of the prophet who cares deeply for the flawed object of his offended passion. Yet there is a simplicity in Shriver's observations on the causes and the remedies for racism. Thus he looks back to Martin Luther King saying in 1961: 'Strangely enough, I can never be what I ought to be, until you are what you ought to be'. This was a truth that Americans all needed to learn, and one that they could learn particularly from an African American understanding of 'the social self'.

While Shriver was attempting to re-invigorate Union, the brief one term in office of Democrat President Jimmy Carter (1976 – 1980) showed that principled liberal Christianity had not died out in political life. Carter was (and still is, in 2021!) a devout Baptist, whose many achievements for social justice have largely been forgotten. But in the

23

wider USA from 1980, the tides of a very different type of Christianity were flowing in, with political implications for the next forty years.

The rise (and rise) of the Christian Right

From the landing of White Puritan settlers 400 years ago, through the colonial period, the founding of the United States and its turbulent history ever since, the life and history of the nation has been intensely shaped by the Christian religion. We might say not that Christianity has 'shaped', but rather that it has *been* the life of the nation, in ways uniquely American. 'One nation under God'.

A kaleidoscopic array of mainly White Protestant believers settled the land that God had given them with all its bounty. For many years they did not doubt either their own rights or their superiority over the Black slaves whom they imported from Africa to increase their wealth and expand their power. White supremacy, too, was often seen as God-given. This is the legacy which has hardly been left behind. Among the many branches of Protestant faith, evangelical revivalism has played a major part, and has had several huge waves of impact and success. Just when other parts of the Western world seemed to be leaving Christianity behind, by the end of the 20th century the USA was embracing a new version of *exceptionalism*, in both faith and politics.

The context and reasons may have varied. Sometimes evangelical fervour has been linked with a particular moral crusade, such as during Prohibition between the world wars, when alcohol was the sin against which battles must be fought. And for the last forty years, opposing abortion has been a motivating and even *the* unifying cause driving a vast movement within conservative religion, both Catholic and Protestant.

One underlying theme is that God's salvation is not of this world. However 'bad' the world or life may be, God gives us a way out, an escape. Which in turn reduces the need for Christian attempts to improve this world.

Another feature is religious fundamentalism, most of all around the Bible. This has fuelled the ongoing resistance to science, or rather to some aspects of scientific research and advance – nearly all Americans, of course, rely on the fruits of scientific and technological progress to enrich their homes and their lives! The most well-known aspect of such resistance is Creationism, along with hostility to or denial of evolution. But fundamentalist religion has also had a deep influence on attitudes to medical advances, as seen recently in vaccine scepticism, and more generally in the denial or dismissal of climate change. The old apocalyptic meme may kick in too: "if God wants to end the world soon by climate chaos or anything else, why should we try and stop Him?"

For many years the Christian Right has been identified as standing for God, guns and the flag. But their gospel is also one of thankfulness for prosperity, and refuge from pain. "I don't come to church to be told what to do, like I'm in school" a complaining elder once told Donald Shriver, "I come here to get comfort". In the end, says revivalist religion (and 'the end' may be soon, very soon, for in extreme cases the 'rapture' is just around the corner) none of that do-gooding matters too much. So too, Freedom is God's greatest gift. Freedom to be who we want to be, not freedom to love our neighbour or live in a better society. Or, as Sarah Palin put it in 2008 when railing against the Obama message: "All that hopey, changey stuff – aren't ya just sick of it?"

This may all be a crude and over-simplified caricature of the Christian Right in modern America, but it's one way of understanding the persistence of racism and the re-emergence of attitudes which had seemed to be on the wane, after the advances and achievements of the civil rights era.

The arrival of Barack Obama as the first Black President in 2009 may have added to the complacent view that conflict in race relations was no longer a threat. Obama was elected, however, not *because* he was Black, but because he offered hope and change. His mixed racial heritage might not have hurt him too much, until Donald Trump fanned the flames of the bi rther conspiracy (spreading the false belief that Obama was not born in the USA). The residual question is to what extent Trump harnessed the racist backlash which was provoked simply by the fact of a Black family residing in the White House for eight years.

The End Times?
There have been many evangelical revivals. But this time round it has

been more overtly political. In 1979, the year in which Jerry Falwell founded the Moral Majority, the television faith healer Pat Robertson effused: "We have, together with the Protestants and the Catholics, enough votes to run the country. And when the people say, 'We've had enough', we are going to take over".

And so, in a sense, in 2016 it came to pass. Except that instead of choosing a man of God, the people elected an outstandingly irreligious and immoral leader, whose deceit and lies have no bounds. This happened with the vast majority of white evangelicals supporting him. They had their reasons, but to be clear, Trump cares little about abortion or the 'pro-life' cause, a top priority for the Christian Right. He appointed strongly conservative justices to the Supreme Court so that he could keep and feed his hold on his political base.

In his ascent to power and his mesmerising, cultic hold on his followers, Trump goaded millions of religious conservatives to embrace the heresy of White Christian nationalism. The key word here is White. All that we might say about the political bias of conservative evangelicals in recent American history applies far more to White than to Black Christians. A clear implication of Make America Great Again is that America can only be great when foreigners, Black people and other minorities are stopped from 'taking over our lives'.

The reasons for the monstrous Trump phenomenon – his success in 2016, almost repeated again in 2020 together with the near-death of American democracy – all this has been endlessly analysed in books and the media. The implications of Trump for the Republican Party, the USA, and the rest of the world, will be with us for years, discussed ad nauseam. The fact that he is no longer President has not stopped his inexhaustible capacity to be the centre of attention and the centre of political influence. No one knows how or when it will all end.

However, Trump's ongoing role in the battle for racial justice, and its intensely political edge, can in 2021 be summed up by the two words: *voter suppression*. The immensely false narrative of a 'stolen election' has resulted in a massive Republican assault on voting rights, across many states, with the aim of derailing the Biden recovery in 2022 and 2024.

The new religious left: Black leaders in the State of Georgia

Democrats have only the slimmest of political advantage in Congress, thanks to the two Democrat Senators for Georgia, one White, one Black, elected early in 2021 as a follow-up to the main 2020 elections. This success would never have happened without years of hard work by one Black woman, a politician named Stacey Abrams, whose parents were two Methodist ministers, and who embodies the classic Black expression of faith and politics in the struggle for justice. She is now a leader of high renown who was among those shortlisted for vice-president by Joe Biden.

It is entirely credible that when standing for Governor of Georgia in 2018, an election she just lost, Stacey Abrams was foiled by the voter suppression tactics of her opponents and the de-registration of hundreds of thousands of legitimate voters in urban and mainly Democrat areas. Still, this did not deflect her from laying the groundwork for the turn-out of minority and low-income voters in 2020. One of the better known features has been 'Souls to the Polls', encouraging Black congregations to complete their Sunday mornings by going straight from church to a polling station. Black churches organize these events throughout the state, evoking the historic experience of enslaved Black people, who only on Sundays might have exercised any token of choice in their lives.

The new Black Senator for Georgia is himself a Pastor: Reverend Raphael Warnock, a graduate with two degrees from, yes, Union Theological Seminary in the City of New York. Here is how he was trailed for a Union series of webinars in April 2021, with the title **Faith and the Fight for a progressive future.**

> Senator Warnock is an unparalleled leader of the religious left. After growing up in public housing, he graduated from Morehouse College and Union to become an ordained minister. He is the youngest person to be selected Senior Pastor at Ebenezer Baptist Church in Atlanta, the former pulpit of Reverend Dr. Martin Luther King.

> Guided by his faith, Sen. Warnock mounted a campaign to become Georgia's first Black senator. He beat the odds and won, despite the gross mischaracterizations of his faith and other attacks. The

right to vote is deeply personal for Sen. Warnock, particularly coming from a state that is notorious for its voter suppression tactics. And as Georgia imposes even more hurdles to voting, Sen. Warnock is fighting for federal legislation to ensure the right to vote is protected and expanded.

This then is the new front for the struggle: to fight the brutal new voting laws. The methods may be modern: economic boycotts, social media organisation and community action. But the energy is in direct line with the cries and songs of the slaves long ago. One of the most striking voting restrictions in Georgia's new elections law is a ban on distributing food and drinks to voters waiting in lines to cast a ballot – even though these waits can, as in 2020, stretch for hours. 'Denying a cup of water to the thirsty' has deep scriptural echoes.

Black church leaders in Georgia and everywhere are nothing if not evangelical and pentecostal. Yet here they rise and protest against restricting the right to vote, because as one pastor puts it '...in the Black church we deal with the whole Black experience'. The arguments for action are steeped in the biblical experience and spiritual lives of generations. These congregations still move to the old stories of liberation and exodus which impel a new kind of struggle today. The suddenness of the new harsh laws enacted in 2021 presents a new, menacing threat.

"I've been to the mountain top" proclaimed Martin Luther King in 1968. "I may not get there with you, but I've seen the Promised Land... and we as a people will get there."

The Promised Land seems once again to be more than another mountain top away. It is a destination which today's Black leaders may have viewed, in faith but not with certainty that they will reach it themselves.

Joe Biden: a liberal, religious president

To commentators in Europe and many younger Democrats in the USA, you can't be a true liberal and religious as well. For decades, the Democratic Party ceded 'faith voters' to the religious right. Joe Biden challenges that view. He is only the second Catholic President in US history, Kennedy being the first. His faith is lifelong and deep. He goes to church on Sundays, and his faith has sustained him unashamedly through the tragedies and trials of his family life.

There is polling evidence that Trump's 2016 hold on the Christian right was weakened by Biden in a state like Wisconsin, where enough Catholics swung over to Biden, just as enough Black and urban voters swung to him in Pennsylvania. Among the often socially conservative Black community, many see a man far more authentically Christian than the Trump who claimed to 'love evangelicals'.

Joe Biden has now re-emphasised his commitment as a man of faith. His inauguration ceremony was full of religious words and choices, as a CNN report observed the day after. On top of the traditional invocation and blessing, *Amazing Grace* was sung. The National Youth Poet Amanda Gorman quoted Micah 4:4 in her dramatic rendition. Biden's own speech kept refering to God and his faith, in a way that no other recent Presidents have done. He quoted from Psalm 30 in a passage about loss and mourning: "Weeping may endure for a night, but joy comes in the morning".

Biden has already tried to encourage greater tolerance and openness across credal differences. He wants to embrace the role that churches, synagogues, mosques and other traditions can play as builders of civil society. He has revived the Office of Faith-Based and Neighborhood Partnerships in the White House. As a 'unifier', he looks for the widest possible range of partnerships against racism and other forms of injustice. This also opens up the chance to win back some of America's religious voters to the side of both freedom and justice.

How can the old dream of a Christian America become a new vision? Martin Luther King's dream – of justice, freedom and peace, as foretold by the prophet Isaiah centuries before Christ – may be faded. But there is at least a glimmer of hope that in all the political and social challenges ahead, religion can cross over from being part of the problem, to being part of the solution.

Edward Cardale is a retired priest in the Diocese of St Albans, and editor of **Crucible.**

Questions for discussion

1. Do you agree that racial injustice is a unique or distinctive evil, or would you prefer it to be seen and addressed alongside other forms of oppression in the world?
2. Which policies for reducing racism do you think are more effective, and how do the churches compare with other social or political organisations in this struggle? How far can a movement such as Black Lives Matter be translated into non-American contexts such as the UK?
3. Is Martin Luther King still a worthy hero in the struggle for racial justice, or would you choose other more recent examples of saintly action on behalf of oppressed peoples?

References

Christian Ethics in Conversation: A Festschrift in honor of Donald W. Shriver Jr., 13th President of Union Theological Seminary in the City of New York. Edited by Isaac B. Sharp and Christian T. Iosso. Cascade Books 2020.

Abrams, Stacey, *Our Time is Now: Power, Purpose and the Fight for a Fair America,* Henry Holt and co. 2020.

Handy, Robert T., *A Christian America: Protestant Hopes and Historical Realities,* O.U.P. 1971

Mead, Walter Russell, *Mortal Splendour:* The American Empire in Transition, Houghton Mifflin 1987

Mekonis, Charles A., With Clumsy Grace: The American Catholic Left 1961 – 1975, The Seabury Press 1979

Shriver, Donald W. Jr., *An Ethic for Enemies: Forgiveness in Politics,* New York O.U.P. 1995

Shriver, Donald W. Jr., *Honest Patriots: Loving a Country enough* to remember its misdeeds, New York O.U.P. 2005

Wills, Gary, *Review Article in the New York Review of Books 20/4/17,* based on *The Evangelicals: The Struggle to Shape America* by Frances FitzGerald

COP 26:
Where lies hope?

STUART ELLIOTT

Climate Change, Hope and the Human Condition is the subtitle of the 2008 book Hell and High Water by theologian Alistair McIntosh. Alistair wrote movingly that he inserted the word 'hope' into the title following the news of his stillborn child: 'It was death's empty glass that did it.'[1] As the father of a neonatal death myself, I can empathise sincerely.

Where do we find hope in the face of a desperate future? Facing the potential scenarios in the IPCC special report SP1.5[2] is traumatic. Central to the Christian message, though, is that new life comes through death. Our glass must first be emptied out.

As I write, the world is still struggling with another year of pandemic restrictions, the like of which we have not seen in our lifetime. In the midst of this, the United Kingdom government is preparing to host the COP26 climate talks this November in Glasgow [COP = UN annual 'Conference of the Parties', the 26th since 1994]. It has pledged an ambitious target of 68% reduction in carbon emissions, but is yet to publish the plan which will enable it to get there. The traumatic truth is that climate change is only one effect of the environmental breakdown that is happening around the world. If ever the glass were empty, if ever we needed hope, surely it is now.

The question remains: in what do we put our hope?

It would be untrue to say that there is no hope in the United Nations

---

[1] McIntosh, Alistair. Hell and High Water, Climate Change, Hope and the Human Condition BIRLINN 2008 p.247

[2] Masson-Delmotte et al (eds). Global Warming of 1.5°C. Intergovernmental Panel on Climate Change Special Report on the impacts of global warming of 1.5°C above pre-industrial levels and related global greenhouse gas emission pathways, in the context of strengthening the global response to the threat of climate change, sustainable development, and efforts to eradicate poverty. Published 2018: https://www.ipcc.ch/sr15/ last accessed 6th June 2021

Crucible October 2021

COP meetings. The signatory nations will meet together this October in China for a COP15 meeting on biodiversity, as well as to prepare for the much-publicised COP26 in November. There is the hope that they will agree binding targets to protect the ecosystem which keeps this planet habitable.

Those who believe the solutions lie with intergovernmental co-operation cite the success of the 1987 Montreal protocol. It was drawn up to eliminate chlorofluorocarbons (CFCs) – the use of which was to blame for the thinning of ozone in the atmosphere.[3] However, environmental breakdown is now all-pervasive. There is no single target for reduction, as there was with CFCs, though carbon (the basic building block of life on earth) is fast becoming the scapegoat of climate change; and the humble plastic bag, once a convenient use of waste oil, is now a scapegoat of environmental breakdown. The UK government prices a plastic bag at 10p[4] but there is, as yet, no similar incentive to reduce the use of other plastics such as bottles. The promised deposit scheme will not be introduced until at least 2024.[5]

Reduction of carbon emissions alone will not solve the planetary ecological breakdown. The eradication of CFC gasses required a technological answer: to find, manufacture and distribute a replacement product. It was a win for the depleted ozone, but it was also a win for the global economy.

In 2019 Greta Thunberg spoke movingly to the UN: 'People are suffering. People are dying. Entire ecosystems are collapsing. We are in the beginning of a mass extinction, and all you can talk about is money and fairy tales of eternal economic growth? How dare you?'[6]

In response to the international agreement made in Paris at COP21 (2015), signatory nations are required to make a pledge for carbon emission reduction ahead of this November's meeting.

---

[3] Lawrence, Matthew. Laybourn-Langton, Laurie. Planet on Fire VERSO 2021 p.86
[4] https://www.bbc.co.uk/news/business-57014762 (Accessed 9th May 2021)
[5] https://www.theguardian.com/environment/2021/mar/24/no-bottle-deposit-return-scheme-for-most-of-uk-until-2024-at-earliest (accessed 13th July)
[6] Thunberg, Greta. Speech given to the UN September 2019

Crucible October 2021

Each year of negotiations sees the window for action narrowing. The speed at which significant actions to reduce carbon emissions and to protect the balance of the planetary ecology will need to be rapid. The IPCC acknowledges the significant global transformation that would be needed for warming limited to 1.5°C[7]. Whether there is the political will is yet another question.

Does the power for real change then solely lie with intergovernmental co-operation? Is there a place for speaking truth to these powers? Perhaps the place to begin is where power truly lies: in the hands of each person to act and to lobby for action. There is hope, and particularly hope in the Christian gospel; for what is still required is an inner transformation.

Three different kinds of hope are currently prevalent:
- Firstly, the hope, or for some the firm belief, that climate change is not happening.
- Secondly, the hope that the technology of the future will fix things.
- Thirdly, the hope that shifting economic activity into areas of sustainable or renewable resources will be *enough* to see us through.

None of these false hopes takes seriously McIntosh's 'empty glass'. Three biblical reflections are offered here in response, which require us to face the painful truth of the global situation, before being able to begin 'to make all things new'. We shall respond to these three kinds of false or inadequate hope.

Hope in denial
The IPCC interim report SR1.5 has high confidence[8] that global temperatures have risen 0.87°c between 1850 and 2015,[9] and that global temperature increases are likely to reach 1.5°c between 2030 and 2050, without rapid and effective action.

It is still possible to hear voices in complete denial of the situation, not least from heavyweight right-wing political figures. Many who

---

[7] IPCC SR15 p52
[8] italics note the particular phrasing of the IPCC reports
[9] McIntosh, Alistair Riders on the Storm BIRLINN 2020 p40

Crucible October 2021

wish to contradict the cautious position of the IPCC and its consensus approach do so by playing down the threat or cherry-picking effects that support their case.

A typical example of these diversionary tactics is the Pacific island of Tuvalu, which is experiencing a net increase in land mass rather than sinking beneath the waves, as had once been forecast.[10] But on a global scale there are many low-lying islands where sea level rise is causing significant issues. The IPCC special report makes it clear that the global mean sea level is rising and accelerating.[11]

For Christians, the Easter promise is that death is not an end: 'Very truly, I tell you, unless a grain of wheat falls into the earth and dies, it remains just a single grain; but if it dies, it bears much fruit.'[12] The hope is that through allowing death, there can be resurrection. A theologically and politically conservative christian position is that this is a disposable planet and humans are simply passing through.[13] This view focuses partly on the promise of restoration 'See, I am making all things new'[14] – strangely welcoming environmental breakdown as a sign of the apocalypse. It looks for the coming Kingdom of God which means a new heaven and earth.[15] This view seems to ignore that what is happening here and now is on God's earth which is blessed by God. It also overlooks the continued covenant relationship in which there is a partnership between God and all of creation. To quote the paraphrase of Revelation 21 in the song by John Bell: 'Behold I make all things new, beginning with you and starting from today.'[16]

This apocalyptic vision is becoming common even in secular writing, in some cases with the welcome acknowledgment that this is a moment of revelation, and – perhaps surprisingly – that we have the power to change our beliefs and actions.

---

[10] https://www.abc.net.au/news/2018-12-19/fact-check-is-the-island-nation-tuvalu-growing/10627318 accessed 7th Jly 2021

[11] Oppenheimer, M. (Et Al): Sea Level Rise and Implications for Low-Lying Islands, Coasts and Communities. In: IPCC Special Report on the Ocean and Cryosphere in a Changing Climate. IN PRESS. 2019 p.323

[12] John 12:24 NRSV

[13] https://theconversation.com/god-intended-it-as-a-disposable-planet-meet-the-us-pastor-preaching-climate-change-denial-147712 (accessed 13th July)

[14] Revelation 21:5 NRSV

[15] cf: Isaiah 65:17, 2 Peter 3:13, Revelation 21:1 NRSV

[16] Bell, John. 'Behold, Behold' in *Come all you People* WILD GOOSE PUBLICATIONS 1995

Crucible October 2021

'In its earlier sense the word 'apocalypse' meant a revelation, an unveiling of things previously unknown. I pray that the revelation which our current apocalypse can bring is the knowledge that we have the power to intervene.'[17]

Denial is a refusal to accept the evidence before us. It is also a denial of the necessary work of internal transformation. Both Thomas and Peter first confront the harsh reality of the death of Jesus with denial, in running away. They are then both confronted with the truth of the resurrection, and make their confession. It would be more honest to be like Thomas ('Unless I see the marks of the nails...'[18]) than Peter, whose triple betrayal is gently absolved over a lakeside breakfast;[19] yet both get to the same point in the end.

This important work of the transformation of the heart can happen only when we are exposed to those with whom we can have compassion, as we identify with their suffering. This means the face-to-face confronting of the truth of nations and peoples whose lives will be irrevocably changed by what is globally happening to our ecosystem. Primarily, this is a privileged western northern hemisphere issue of justice; and we in these nations are indebted to organisations like Christian Aid who enable these exposures of truth in their Climate Justice campaigning.

For Christians, it means allowing the Kingdom of God to come though the revelation of Jesus, who brings restoration and healing, by the transformation of one heart at a time. This is truly hopeful, for it relies not on out-of-reach political policy or technology, but on person-to-person conversation, compassion and revelation. Once the heart is changed, the actions follow. If the grain of wheat dies, it bears much fruit.

Hope in a techno-fix

"We've got the technology, we just need to use it" is a phrase that is heard often. Yet many are putting their hope in technological solutions that have not yet been shown to work effectively at scale, or that use

[17] Macdonald, Helen. Vesper Flights JONATHAN CAPE 2020 p.64
[18] John 20.24ff NRSV
[19] John 21.15ff NRSV

Crucible October 2021

huge amounts of energy in order to 'solve' the problem of burning fossil fuels.

Carbon capture and storage can mimic the effects of trees and plants which scrub carbon from the atmosphere, preventing it from mixing with oxygen to create CO_2. There is much hope that technical solutions will be able to mitigate the worst emissions which are drivers of climate change. The IPCC states that 'all pathways to limit global warming to 1.5°C, with limited or no overshoot, project the use of carbon dioxide removal (CDR) in the order of 100-1000 billion tons of CO_2 over the 21st century.'[20]

Yet the danger with putting our hope in new technology is that the next best thing is always just around the corner.[21] CDR will use a colossal amount of energy, which needs to be produced without releasing significantly more carbon. We've created a hole by 'shovelling carbon out of the ground and into the sky. The first thing to do is stop shovelling. All CCS [Carbon Capture and Storage] does is take teaspoons out of massive scoops of carbon and puts them back in the hole.'[22] Whilst the planting of trees is important for carbon storage and soil stability, particularly the mycorrhizal networks, vastly more important is their safeguarding for the future, ending mass deforestation and biodiversity loss. It is clear that technology and natural solutions will need to be taken together. Most importantly, this means that we cannot rely solely on the solutions of the future. There is a need to face our situation humbly, and reduce the amount of energy we are currently consuming. Collective efforts need to be taken at all levels to strengthen the global response to climate change. It really is down to us.[23]

The dilemma for us is: where do we put our energy when there are so many areas that need our advocacy and action? As Christians we may hope to have the humility to listen to the voices of those who are at the

---

[20] IPCC, 2018: Summary for Policymakers. In: Global Warming of 1.5°C. An IPCC Special Report on the impacts of global warming of 1.5°C above pre-industrial levels and related global greenhouse gas emission pathways, in the context of strengthening the global response to the threat of climate change, sustainable development, and efforts to eradicate poverty Masson-Delmotte, et al(eds.). In Press. p17

[21] Mann p.150ff

[22] Mann p.153

[23] McIntosh 2020 p80

COP 26: Where lies hope?

frontline of the ecological breakdown.

Whilst teaching his disciples, Jesus puts a child among them.[24] In this beautiful interaction between Jesus, a child and the disciples, he shows up the human capacity for humility; but also for ignoring the voices of those we feel we can speak over. Interestingly, this comes in a passage where the disciples are arguing about who is the greatest. Jesus says two things. Firstly that a childlike humility is essential; and secondly, that welcoming a child is a sign of welcoming Jesus and God himself. Jesus clearly had an understanding of how a child viewed the world, and how the world viewed children.

Essentially it comes to putting ourselves to one side, and viewing the world as a child might: this is the difficult work of kenosis. To be emptied of pride and ego, to be able to see truly without prejudice, is the vision of Paul in his letter to the Philippians. This requires self-sacrifice in learning to be humble in the face of the earth. In her book 'Blessed are the Consumers', lifelong campaigner for eco-feminism and justice Sallie McFague argues that we need to accept our mortality for the sake of the whole of humanity and the planet.

> 'Is it enough to imagine another model for abundant living: one in which, by identifying ourselves with all others (the universal self), we can accept our own biological death, knowing, as Dorothea Soelle puts is, that "this creation ... remains alive"? By itself this may not be enough, in which case our prospects and the prospects of a just, sustainable planet are in serious jeopardy.'[25]

Hope in constant growth

The hope that there is no empty glass, and the hope that some technical miracle will mitigate our emissions, are both underwritten by a third and more polluting hope: in the economic model of capitalism.

Consumer spending is reliant on the availability of goods and services, which are in turn reliant on the raw materials used in production. The extraction of a large proportion of these, including fossil fuels, is

---

[24] Matthew 18.1ff NRSV; see also Mark 9.33ff NRSV
[25] McFague p165

Crucible October 2021

precisely what is doing an awful lot of harm to the planetary ecological balance. Natural capital is not currently taken into account on the balance sheet though there are some bold propositions.

The Montreal protocol on CFCs was successful because it relied on this capitalist world-view to solve the problem. In order to maintain growth, death cannot be allowed to have a place. An empty glass is not an option; consumer spending must not diminish. One example of this is the drive towards electric cars. Changing the fuel of private transport from direct fossil-fuel-driven engines to stored energy in electric batteries is a solution which raises more questions than it answers. It is true that the direct emissions from driving the vehicle are low, for electric vehicles. They cannot be zero due to consumables such as tyres and brakes. This might improve the air quality of congested roads in cities, but it does little to tackle global carbon emissions, unless the source of the electricity is also low carbon. And all this, before even thinking about the production of the car, or the mining of rare earth minerals for the batteries, which is a complex ethical discussion in its own right.[26] The only true winner here is the economy.

Until we are able to ensure that the economy works to sustain the Earth, rather than to maintain financial growth, schemes such as carbon trading or a carbon tax will have little impact. It has been suggested that a tax targeted directly on those who are extracting the carbon may be the simplest solution.[27] Both pollution and subsequent clean-up operations raise GDP, and are therefore seen as positive economic drivers. But the current economic system, where all growth is good, and natural capital is not accounted for, cannot work to mitigate the complex environmental breakdown we are facing.

Hope in changed hearts – a more radical vision

Christians are not immune to the financial world. Almost every church has investments in financial institutions. Though 'negative' ethical investment policies (avoiding investment in damaging activities) limit the scope of investing, we need to learn to put our money where our faith is. Jesus' critique of the financial world doesn't come any

---

[26] Berners-Lee p99ff

[27] Berners-Lee p146

stronger than in Myers and DeBode's reading of the parable of the talents.

> '[Jesus'] pedagogic purpose was twofold: to unmask the illusions his audience had about the status quo and their place in it, and then to help that audience open its heart and mind to what he proposed as an alternative – what he called the "kingdom of God."'[28]

In this parable, Jesus is particularly critical of the financial dealings of the empire. The transformative moment is when the so-called 'untrustworthy slave' buries the master's money in the ground. This action shows up the true worth of the coin: on its own the coin cannot give growth, and certainly cannot produce a crop that can be harvested. When the master calls in the investments, he replies to this third slave that he ought to have at least invested it with the bankers so that the master could have what was rightfully his. This shows up the arrogance of the investment: expecting to reap a reward simply because the money was invested, and the investor doing nothing to bring about the return. 'You knew, did you, that I reap where I did not sow, and gather where I did not scatter?'[29]

Myers and DeBode reflect that slavery in this parable is to the financial empire. Even the slaves who are congratulated for their returns are still in slavery – only with more responsibility to create even greater wealth for the master.

Churches have been encouraged recently to divest from fossil fuels by, for example, the charity Operation Noah.[30] This divestment is a clear signal that fossil fuels are not the future of energy – or even, in these turbulent times, a reliable source of investment income. A more radical vision still is required: 'Sadly, our churches no longer embrace a radical vision of history that chooses the power of Jesus over and against the power of empire.'[31]

---

[28] Towering Trees and Talented Slaves: Jesus Parables
by Ched Myers and Eric DeBode
From The Other Side Online, © 1999 The Other Side, May-June 1999, Vol. 35, No. 3.
[29] Matthew 25:26 NRSV
[30] https://operationnoah.org/news-events/news/press-release-faith-institutions-divest-from-fossil-fuels-and-call-for-just-recovery-ahead-of-g7-and-cop26/

Crucible October 2021

We need to put our money where our faith is. If our faith is in the restorative power of Jesus, and in the vision of the Kingdom of God built on the unconditional love which we endeavour to reflect, then our financial investments should follow those guiding principles, rather than seeking a return at any cost.

Financially, this would mean using our investments positively, rather than negatively. It might mean taking a much smaller financial return, but measuring growth in terms of wellbeing and positive outcomes. There are already many alternative investment opportunities for those who want to invest in community and social projects. The Kindling Trust, run by Helen Woodcock and Chris Walsh, operates one such project in Manchester. Funding for the Kindling Farm project came through Ethex, an alternative investment platform where investors can 'make money do good'.[32] Our hope lies in communities supported by grassroots organisations such as The Kindling Trust, whose whole focus is on people and the planet.

COP26 *could* be a gear-change meeting, as was COP21 in Paris. But while these international meetings offer a pathway and make legislation possible, the power for change lies squarely with individuals and communities: in hearts and humility. With hope placed firmly in changed and humble hearts, and with a vision of the kingdom of God which truly values each individual rather than financial worth, the possibility is that positive choices for the future of the planet will be taken. ' "Hope is a good thing, maybe the best of things." Alone it won't solve this problem. But drawing upon it, we will'.[33]

The opportunity is ours to grasp.

Stuart Elliott is a priest in the Church in Wales, ministering in the benefice of Bro Gwydyr in Snowdonia. He is a member of the Church in Wales' national environmental steering group, and has been instrumental in achieving the commitment of the Church to reach net carbon zero by 2030, and in participation in A Rocha's Eco Church and Eco Diocese scheme.

[31] Myers, DeBode.
[32] https://www.ethex.org.uk/invest/kindling-farm
[33] Mann p.267

References

Bell, John, 'Behold, Behold' in *Come all you People*, Wild Goose Publications 1995

Berners-Lee. Mike, There is no Planet B, C.U.P 2019

Davey, Edward, *Given Half a Chance*, Unbound 2019

IPCC reports available at www.ipcc.ch

Lawrence, Matthew, and Laybourn-Langton, Laurie, *Planet on Fire* Verso 2021

Macdonald, Helen, *Vesper Flights, Jonathan Cape 2020*

McFague, Sallie, *Blessed are the Consumers*, Fortress 2013

McIntosh, Alistair, *Hell and High Water*, Birlinn 2008

McIntosh, Alistair, *Riders on the Storm*, Birlinn 2020

Mann, Michael E, The New Climate War, Scribe 2021

Myers, Ched and DeBode, Eric, *Towering Trees and Talented Slaves: Jesus Parables.*

From The Other Side Online, © 1999 The Other Side, May-June 1999, Vol. 35, No. 3.

Geopolitics and Human Identity

STEPHEN GREEN

We live at a dangerous moment in history. When China overtakes America as the largest economy in the world – as it will do sometime in the next few years – that will just be a milestone. The best central forecast for China's growth is that it will continue at a reasonable pace for the next generation. Sheer size therefore means that it will not just be the largest *but a long way* the largest economy in the world. Its influence – already expanding rapidly – will become ever greater. China is here to stay.

But so is America. Some have depicted this great chess game as one which has already been lost and won. But they are wrong. It may look as though one of the players has a single mind looking several moves ahead all the time, while the other moves capriciously and without any apparent or consistent strategy. But we shouldn't be deceived by the dysfunctional short-termism of Washington politics. The system was set up to be gridlocked – and much of the time it is. Yet the incredible inventiveness and dynamism of American society will ensure that it is the counteracting force China has to reckon with, for as far ahead as any of us can foresee. Most chess games result in a winner; but not all. This one is more likely to end in a stalemate.

A contest of political ideologies – or is it about something deeper?

The Marxist rhetoric of today's Chinese Communist Party is no more than skin deep. Mao used the language of Marxism; but it did not fit Chinese circumstances any more than it had been relevant to a highly rural and backward Russia. And in any event, China's urban transformation has achieved most of its momentum and economic success only after Mao, by which time the Chinese Communist Party was openly talking of 'socialism with Chinese characteristics' and pursuing a policy of economic flexibility which owed more to Adam Smith than to anything that could be described as authentically Marxist.

What lies thinly concealed by that rhetoric is a very different version of the relationship between the state, society and the individual. China's ruling party has become a motherland party, of a kind that is in fact familiar from the twentieth century. And indeed, we should focus not only on China but on other major nations of the modern world: something is at work in many of them which modern Europeans tend to underestimate. For in country after country, there is a rising cultural self-assertiveness – echoing, in some ways, the overweening nationalism of the Europe of the nineteenth century. China's Communist Party has its basis as a motherland party in the pervasive patriotism which is almost tangible on the streets and in the social media of modern China. Others seek to tap analogous cultural roots too.

The implications of such cultural assertion are significant. The Western powers have tended to assume that at their best they stand for core values which have been hard won through history *and which are universal in their implications*. The West takes the view that these values are the heritage of a shared history of religious struggle, of philosophical reflection and of scientific exploration which laid the foundations of modernity. It is an odyssey which involved tortuous twists and turns as well as terrible blood-letting. But Europeans and Americans have wanted to believe that what has emerged is something profoundly important for the whole world of the twenty first century.

In the European version of this narrative, the universal values include: a commitment to rationalism, democracy, human rights, the rule of law, equality and fairness, social compassion and toleration. America has been on a similar *but not the same journey*. For the centre of gravity of the American identity is in fact crucially different from that of Europe. America may no longer be young enough to claim innocence. But it is still in an important sense the New World which left the old behind. Even now, America is a country of immense space, with a population density much lower than in the crowded heartlands of Europe and Asia. And somehow, that space still translates into a sense of potential: the individual can always move on.

The myths of America are onward-looking, forward-looking. Alexis de Tocqueville, the perceptive French aristocrat who visited the country in 1831, noticed a special sense of purpose, even calling. He traced a distinctive American identity to its point of departure – the Puritanism of New England. Tocqueville wrote that this 'was not just a religious doctrine: in many respects it shared the most absolute democratic and republican theories', as a result of 'two perfectly distinct elements which elsewhere have often been at war with one another but which in America it was somehow possible to incorporate with each other, forming a marvellous combination: the *Spirit of Religion and the Spirit of Freedom.*'

This New World is older than it was, and has known the pain of civil war, the shame of slavery and traumatic failure in Vietnam - as well as a gnawing sense of dissatisfaction with more recent unhappy excursions in the Middle East. It sees its strategic interests as threatened by the rise of China, and is gradually coming to recognise that its time as the world's only superpower has drawn to a close. The adjustment will be painful.

Europe too has had to learn about the loss of former glory. But America and Europe are different, not only because their geopolitical position and interests are different but because their history is different; and this means that their identities are different. Europeans share much with America, of course. At one level, both Europeans and Americans are inheritors of Christendom and of the Enlightenment. But at another level there are obvious and profound differences in values and priorities. America is more individualistic than the Europeans (even whilst also being more patriotic). This is the legacy of Locke, of that Puritanism which de Tocqueville remarked on, and of the millions of Eurasian immigrants who arrived in the nineteenth and twentieth centuries - whose energy and determination were certainly not captured by the image of 'the tired, the poor and the huddled masses yearning to be free' (from the lines by Emma Lazarus which are quoted on the Statue of Liberty). America has a flexibility and a dynamism, shown in an economy which is constantly reinventing itself in unexpected ways.

But other voices are now questioning the universality of America's liberal democratic order. East Asians in particular question the effectiveness of messy, short-termist democracy. South Asian thinkers question the materialism and individualism into which modern western societies seem to descend. And many in Muslim communities question the secularism which seems to attack their understanding of family values. Moreover, throughout the world many have felt a revulsion at the inequality which has seemed to be its inevitable concomitant; and many have bridled at the transactional individualism and the materialist implication that the value of everything is reflected in its price.

This points to an uncomfortable possibility: *that there may be cultural differences deep enough to put in question whether there are universal ideas or values at all.*

A dialectic of human self-understanding...

In other words, the contest between America and China is not just about political ideology. It is much deeper: it is a contest of world views. The American world view sets the inalienable subjectivity of the self at its core. It is encapsulated in those great watchwords of the founders of America: 'life, liberty and the pursuit of happiness'. By contrast, the great alternative on the world stage of this century – the Confucian-infused culture which is the bedrock of the Chinese world view – is not primarily focussed on the autonomy of the self. It sees the individual in a wider familial, social and even cosmic context; so it has less to say about rights but much to say about position, purposes and obligations in life.

In fact, the fundamental issue is about human self-understanding: at the end of the day, are we individuals who make what we can of the world we find ourselves in? Or do we have a place in an order of things which somehow imposes responsibilities on us? The individualistic American world view answers an emphatic yes to the first question; the Chinese world view answers an equally instinctive yes to the second.

Few would want to argue that either side of this debate has all the good arguments and has nothing to learn from the other. *And neither is intrinsically more Christian than the other.* This means that the debate needs to be a dialogue. What matters to us all is whether those two world views can somehow be dovetailed as the human odyssey continues over the rest of this century. Each has a very long trail of history and thought behind it, and neither is likely to prevail over the other in the geopolitics of the coming decades. The outcome of this dialogue matters for the peace of nations; it matters for the growth of the human spirit; it matters for successful economic and social development; it matters for trustful commerce; and it matters for the sustainability of life on our fragile planet.

That engagement, if it to be enriching on both sides, has to range over a broad agenda. It should not surrender the right to moral discourse. But it does need to explore the specific histories that shape identity. It should explore the aesthetic expression of human life experience down the ages in visual arts, in music, in poetry. It should explore the way metaphysics has sought to make sense of things at the most general level. It needs to understand the values that have their underpinnings in such metaphysics. Above all, it needs to explore the way human identity and its relationship to the 'other' is understood.

...and a possible basis for hope

There is a possible basis for hope in the face of this challenge. For there are strands of thought from classical antiquity in both the Chinese, Greek and Abrahamic thought worlds which are as relevant today as they ever were. *These themes suggest that there is indeed a basis for convergence between the Chinese and American world views, as humanity confronts the challenges of the modern age.*

The first point to note is there are remarkable resonances between Confucius and Aristotle on the virtues that are conducive to and manifested in the good life. They define the good life differently: for Aristotle it is *eudaimonia*, for Confucius it is *the Way* that is the focus. Aristotle's *eudaimonia* is best translated perhaps as wellness of spirit, though it is often translated as happiness (the pursuit of which is an 'inherent and inalienable right' enshrined in America's founding Declaration of Independence, but which can all too easily evaporate into something more superficial and transient). Confucius draws on the central concept of Chinese metaphysics: the Way is an image very deeply embedded in Chinese thought from its earliest stirrings. For Laozi it was the origin of all things, prior both logically and causally to both heaven and earth, ineffable, and defying categorisation as either being or non-being. But Confucius set a trend which later became the mainstream: for *The Analects* the Way is the way of heaven, which is *immanent in human experience* as the principle of moral behaviour (rather than a transcendent influence on it).

The Chinese tradition, with Confucius as a formative representative, prefers to merge what Aristotelianism keeps more distinct. For the Chinese instinct, the ultimate principle is to be found within experience (sometimes within nature, as later Europeans, notably Spinoza, would also do, but more prominently, as in Confucius, Mencius and Xunzi, in human nature). By contrast, for classical Greece, the ultimate source of worth and of virtue lies in the realm of the transcendent. This became even more unambiguous later on, in the guise of mediaeval Christian, Islamic and Jewish philosophy.

Given that profound difference and all its many implications, it is all the more striking that the two perspectives come to focus, in a somewhat similar way, on living well by acting through an appropriate sense of benevolent purpose. The Chinese concept is *'ren'* - often translated as 'benevolence' but perhaps better, because more comprehensively, as 'humanity'; the classical European thought world similarly recognised that *eudaimonia* requires behaviour towards the 'other' which is humane and hence virtuous.

In both cases, there is an intimate connection between benevolence/ humanity and another key concept - justice/rightness. The concept of justice also has very deep roots in both thought worlds; it recognises what is 'due' to the 'other' (where the 'other' may include the gods, as in Homer). For Plato, justice underpins the rational order; for Aristotle justice is determined by what is fair as well as wha t the law of the *polis* determines; for Aquinas it is ordained by divinely ordered natural law. And in China, the concepts of *ren* and of *yi* (justice/rightness) have been linked as a pair from early Confucianism onwards (one of the earliest usages being in The *Doctrine of the Mean*, one of the four books making up the canon of Confucianism and traditionally attributed to Confucius's grandson).

But this begs a question in both cases. Just how far does the requirement for humanity/benevolence and for justice/rightness in social interaction extend? Is it to family? to one's 'kind' (to use an English term rich in connotations of family or clan connection as well as of good will)? Is it to humanity at large ('kind' in its very broadest sense)? Or is it to all sentient beings and indeed to the natural environment as a whole?

This question has received different answers at various times from different voices within the Chinese tradition. One of the major points of contention between the Confucian and Mohist traditions was precisely about the issue of the universality of moral obligation. It was the practical realism of Confucius which prevailed; to use Adam Smith's terminology, the degree of 'sympathy' gets weaker, the more distant the relationship (with distance being based primarily on the degree of kinship - thus, family is closest, the species is furthest). In Europe, such an explicit focus on kinship was less prominent; but the moral distance between near and far is as evident in Aristotle (for whom the *polis* set the bounds of obligation), in the Hebrew distinction between neighbour and foreigner, in the praxis of Christendom (notwithstanding the radical redefinition of the *neighbour* in the New Testament parable of the Good Samaritan) and in the Islamic distinction between the ummah and the world beyond.

It is important to recognise that in both cases thought patterns were far from monolithic. In China, for example, there was a long running contest of ideas about the Way. In particular, it is worth noting that Zhuangzi represents a view that the human Dao is just part of a dominant Dao of nature. Such a perspective tends to play down the metaphysical significance and moral importance of human agency and indeed risks a quietism about human activity of any sort. Xunzi, who flourished in the third century BCE, and who stands in the Confucian tradition, is highly critical both of this Daoist perspective of Zhuangzi and also of the optimist humanism of Mencius. For Xunzi, in contrast to Zhuangzi, the dominant Dao is the human Dao; but in contrast to Mencius, human nature is a mix of reason, emotion and potentially destructive desires. In its natural state, human psychology risks being captured by desires which have physical bases but which can never be adequately sated; human reason thus becomes a calculation of how best to sate the desire. The way out of this entrapment is to inculcate into this natural psychology the powers and virtues that come through learning and are nourished through appropriate ritual - *and chief of which is the power of benevolence*. Thus Xunzi articulates a metaphysics in which the seeds of a positivist but realist role for human creativity and self-transformation can be detected.

The optimism of the eighteenth century (detectable in Chinese as well as in European thought) has of course been replaced in the twenty first century by a much clearer recognition of the damage the human species is doing to itself in its headlong rush into modernity. And as we seek firmer, common ground, we shall be challenged more and more insistently by these venerable principles of charity and equity - benevolence and justice - ren and yi. Both concepts have to be expanded in scope well beyond anything the medieval world understood, and also well beyond what we have been used to in the last two centuries. In particular, it is necessary to see these principles extended and applied trans-generationally, if we are successfully to meet the challenges of climate change and environmental degradation.

But they have the capacity to be thus extended. And because they play such a key role in both the two major cultural traditions we have been discussing, they are therefore the basis for that convergent dialogue which is now so urgent. The dialogue will be hard for both traditions, because these principles challenge the comfortable assumptions of each; and they do so from within. The full meaning of ren and yi is a standing critique of the Chinese geopolitical world view; the full meaning of benevolence and the right is equally a standing critique of the American ideology. It is almost as if neither protagonist needs to do more than to invite the other to look in the mirror of their own principles. If they do so, they can hardly avoid seeing the beam in their own eye.

Worlds apart – or not?
I end with two quotations which it may seem surprising and even provocative to juxtapose. For all the profound and obvious differences of context and of metaphysical belief, there is a distinct and fascinating echo between the two.

The first is from Dong Zhongshu, a Confucian scholar of the second century BC, who wrote in a text known as 'Luxuriant Gems of the Spring and Autumn Annals':

What is meant by ren? Ren is loving others with compassion, living in concord...it has no mind to hurt or wrong others; it has no will to scheme behind someone else's back...It has no desire to make others sad. It does not engage in backbiting or flattery. It does not act against others. Therefore its mind is at ease; its will is at peace...its desires moderated; its affairs easy; its conduct according to the Way.

The second is from Saint Paul's famous purple passage on love/charity, written about two hundred years later:

> Love is patient, love is kind, it does not envy, it does not boast, it is not proud. It does not dishonour others, it is not self-seeking, it is not easily angered, it keeps no record of wrongs. Love does not delight in evil, but rejoices in the truth. It always protects, always trusts, always hopes, always perseveres.

Setting these two quotations alongside each other is not to suggest that there are not important differences between the concept of *ren* as used by Dong Zhongshu and the *agape* of Saint Paul. But it is to argue that the instinct of love is a deep human universal. We all know that reconciling the messy global realities of power and self-interest with this human yearning, and all that it implies, will never be easy. But we can at least recognise what is common to all humanity, find hope in it, and draw inspiration for the dialogue we know we must have in the coming decades.

> *Stephen Green was the Chairman of HSBC, and Minister of State for Trade and Investment in the Coalition Government. He is also an Anglican priest. He has written several books, including 'The Human Odyssey: East, West and the Search for Universal Values' (SPCK, 2019), on which this article is based.*

For further exploration: see an accessible and comprehensive introduction to classical Chinese metaphysical debate, in 'Disputers of the Tao: Philosophical Argument in Ancient China' by A.C.Graham (Open Court Publishing, 2003).

Forum

Law without coercion: exhortation and doctrine in the canon law of the Church of England

RUSSELL DEWHURST

St Thomas Aquinas famously defines law as 'an ordinance of reason for the common good, made by him who has care of the community, and promulgated' (ST I-II, Q90 a4). His definition does not mention coercion, but in a world where people are not perfectly virtuous, Aquinas admits that law must necessarily be coercive. This coercive nature of law has been brought to the fore of the public mind during the Coronavirus Pandemic. To reduce the spread of the disease, we have been told what we should and should not do by means of both guidance and law. Guidance is accompanied by no direct legal sanction. Where a particular restriction is law, on the other hand, there is a threat of sanctions (e.g. fines for gathering with a certain number of people).

In the canon law of the Church of England, by contrast, there are canons which carry no threat of sanction. The canons are just one part of the ecclesiastical law of the Church of England, and in their current form they date substantially from the 1960s, with subsequent amendment and addition. Many of the canons concern the obligations of the clergy, and these obligations can be enforced by means including the Clergy Discipline Measure and capability procedure. But there are others which do not admit of any enforcement, and this, as we have seen, seems unexpected in a body of law.

Most strikingly, there are canons whose purposes seem entirely doctrinal or hortatory. Doctrinal canons have a purely teaching function, e.g. on the sign of the cross at baptism (canon B25). Hortatory canons assert a duty on lay church members to do something, but there is no legal penalty or sanction for failing to do so e.g. the duty to seek to heal schisms (canon A8). In this respect, such canons might seem more akin to the Coronavirus guidance discussed above, rather than law as such, yet they are included in the canons cheek by jowl alongside enforceable law.

Even in the case of clergy, many canons can in theory be enforced by clergy discipline, but in practice are enforced primarily by community expectation or by individual conscience: for example, the obligation of the clergy to say daily the Morning and Evening Prayer (canon C26).

Why, then, should there be provisions in a body of law which are not enforced by sanction? Would we not gain clarity by removing all doctrinal and hortatory canons and converting them into 'guidance' as in the secular Coronavirus example above? I do not think so, and I have come to appreciate the presence of these canons very much. I offer the following five reasons for why we should cherish the doctrinal and hortatory canons:

Firstly, there is long-standing historical precedent. The great 20th century canonist Bishop Eric Kemp traced this tradition from the early church, through the 17th century Anglican canons, to the present day. Writing in his 1956 Introduction to Canon Law he said, 'Much of canon law has always been concerned with the norms of conduct, and has indicated standards which the church thought ought to be observed but was not prepared to enforce by action at law.'

Secondly, the church's teaching and exhortation takes on a different character, and an added weight, by virtue of its presence in the canons. The church has relatively few documents which are 'constitutional', that is official, slow to change, enduring over a long period, and constitutive of our self-understanding. The 16th and 17th century Anglican formularies do not readily admit of addition. Authorised liturgies are an important source of self-understanding under the principle of *lex orandi, lex credendi,* but the kind of teaching which can be incorporated in the liturgy is tightly-drawn. The General Synod can pass resolutions, but it seems to me that while such resolutions can respond nimbly to the questions of the day, they do not usually have an enduring 'constitutional' nature. When a teaching takes its place in the canons, however, it does take on a unique character and becomes part of the church's identity.

We can take, as an example, Canon DA1. Section DA has only been added to the canons in the past couple of years, and deals with religious communities in the Church of England. Canon DA1 is a doctrinal canon: it is a statement on religious life which affirms the Church of England's belief that, for example, those whose lives are marked by consecrated celibacy, poverty, and obedience are responding to God's call. This is significant, given the Church of England's history that includes the dissolution of monasteries in the 16th century and the controversies connected with their return since the 19th century. The inclusion of this statement in the church's canons, therefore, gives this once-controversial teaching a very formal, enduring, and constitutional character that it would not have if contained solely in a report or resolution of some church body.

Thirdly, the presence of doctrinal and hortatory canons gives a 'completeness' to the subjects covered by the canons. Canon law is, at heart, applied theology. It is concerned with how we live out our Christian faith and how we understand our life as church. The canons, therefore, would stand as incomplete without provisions relating to spiritual duties to God and neighbour. Receiving communion, examining one's conscience, observing Sunday – these are ecclesial duties for all Christians, not just clergy, and are rightly so described in the canons. But the canonical expression of these duties are norms and standards, more suited to inculcation through the church's pastoral ministry than enforcement by the court. A central purpose of law is, of course, to protect rights, and it must be able to resort to coercion to do so. But law is also a school that directs us to live in a certain way; and it is with this purpose in mind that canon law teaches, exhorts, and encourages.

Fourthly, the presence of doctrinal canons, whose sole purpose is to teach, points us to the teaching function of every canon. Other community rules, such as the Rule of Benedict, have frequently been found to be worthwhile subjects of study, group discussion, and commentary. The canons too are eminently suitable for study. In 2020, the Ecclesiastical Law Society ran Zoom reading groups over a period of nine months. Clergy, lawyers, academics, and other church members discussed the canons, their theological roots, historical background, legal effects, and ecumenical equivalents. The fact that so many stayed the course is testament to the richness of what we found in our reading together. In 2021, a dozen reading groups across the Anglican Communion are studying the *Principles of Canon Law Common to the Church of the Anglican Communion,* which further underlines the potential of canon law to deepen theological understanding and

Crucible October 2021

ecclesial identity.

Fifthly, and finally, we might even argue that the presence of doctrinal and hortatory provisions in the law of the Church points to her self-understanding as a divine society. Aquinas thought that in a community of the perfectly virtuous – a community of saints – there would be law, but there would not be coercion. By the inclusion of a select category of canons which teach and exhort non-coercively, the church's law is eschatologically ordered, anticipating the life of the Kingdom, and assisting each member voluntarily to act in love – which is the fulfilling of the law.

Russell Dewhurst is a PhD student in canon law at Cardiff University and assistant priest of St Mary's, West Chiltington.

Russell Dewhurst and Stephen Coleman are currently working on a commentary on the canons of the Church of England, intended for publication in the near future.

Book Reviews

Hospitality, Service, Proclamation: Interfaith Engagement as Christian Discipleship

Tom Wilson
SCM Press, 2019, 192pp, pbk, £19.99

Interfaith engagement is an area of ministry which all too often becomes a battleground for other theological sensitivities. This is sometimes due to interfaith engagement being relegated to a secondary status within Christian discipleship. Tom Wilson's book offers an important corrective to such ingrained assumptions. His aim is to show the reader that there are Christian ways of doing interfaith work (p. vii) and that interfaith activity is 'a Christian course of action' (1).

Wilson's argument rests on three themes: hospitality, service, and proclamation. Throughout, Wilson notes the tension that exists between these but demonstrates 'how they provide a framework for interfaith engagement as a form of Christian discipleship' (2).

The first chapter sets forth a rationale for Christian engagement in interfaith activity. Wilson explores some of the obstacles that prevent Christians from engaging in such activity. He sensitively tackles one such perceived obstacle, namely the Christian calling to mission and evangelism. He prefers the term 'intentional growth' (p. 15). Wilson draws on examples from other religious traditions to demonstrate that such an expansive concern is not unique to Christians. He then gives four examples of how interfaith engagement has strengthened his own Christian faith. Each of these is offered in the form of a question raised in the course of interfaith engagement with a particular community. Opportunities to 'pause' throughout this chapter and the book as a whole are especially helpful for those reading this as part of a church-wide reflection or reading group.

A second chapter explores the well worn typology of Christian approaches to other faiths: inclusivism, exclusivism, and pluralism. An introductory literature review offers a series of excellent examples of thinkers who can be broadly classified according to each of these positions. Wilson presents these different approaches to allow the reader to think through their own position more clearly without forcing a particular opinion (p. 53). His closing remarks on the difficulty of categorising individual approaches according to this typology are particularly helpful for students approaching this subject for the first time. Likewise, his ordering of the literature review - placing pluralism first - helps the reader take seriously Christian thinkers who advocate this minority option, which is often too quickly passed over by the majority positions of exclusivism and inclusivism. Students sometimes struggle to comprehend how Christians have entertained pluralism in a theologically rigorous way, and Wilson's presentation is a helpful resource for students wishing to critique this position fairly.

Wilson's next chapter offers a survey of Biblical material on interfaith engagement. This chapter is especially useful for those thinking through how to preach on the subject of interfaith engagement, or to resource Bible studies or home groups. Wilson shows that whilst sometimes the Bible's witness in this area is reduced to proclamation, there are many examples within Scripture that 'support the importance of offering hospitality to people of all faiths and none, and of acts of selfless service' (85).

The final chapters are perhaps the most practical, focussing on when and how Christian interfaith engagement might take place. The first explores the different settings in which interfaith engagement might occur and is organised in 'five broad categories: church, school, other places of worship, the home, and the public square ' (113). Reading through the examples in this chapter helps the reader imagine where in their own context opportunity for interfaith engagement may arise. The chapter on 'how' such engagement can take place offers further examples which can help the reader reflect on their own potential contribution to interfaith engagement as a disciple of Christ. Wilson's conclusion to this chapter summarises some of the key themes of the book. He argues that this area of discipleship requires security of faith but offers great opportunity for learning and growth. In doing so, Wilson invites the reader 'to remain alert to the tension between service, proclamation and hospitality, as both guest and host. All are important elements of the Christian faith, and no one element can be prioritised at the expense of the others' (139).

For Wilson, discernment is vital. Each context will require a different balance of emphasis between service, proclamation, and hospitality. Wilson's book is an important invitation to this task of discipleship which is to discern how we are called to exercise service, proclamation, and hospitality in our varying contexts.

An appendix containing practical wisdom and advice on how to

Crucible October 2021

engage with particular faith communities will be especially welcome to those engaging with different faith communities as they move into new areas of ministry or encounter a particular faith community anew. This book is a welcome tool to all such fresh encounters and the Christian calling to provide hospitality, to serve, and to proclaim.

Simon Cuff, St. Mellitus College, London

Shame and the Church: Exploring and Transforming Practice
Sally Nash
SCM Press, 2020, 193pp, pbk, £19.99

Sally Nash's avowed focus in this book is mainly on 'the shame we don't deserve' (3, quoting Smedes). She has been studying shame in the church for a decade, and much of the book examines a range of exclusionary dynamics in the western church which are experienced by individuals as occasions of shaming. Wonderfully, she begins the journey from an experience of shame by her eight-year-old self, and allusions to this pop up lightly but poignantly at intervals through the book.

The main new data source for the book is a set of 312 questionnaire responses from church leaders, church members and theological educators, mainly in British or American churches. This produces a clear focus on the experience of shaming in the context of a local church or other Christian institution.

The testimonies from people who have experienced shame in the church are often vivid and thought-provoking, such as: 'People who minister can be a right pain in the backside. I do not need ministry; I need love' (130). Many times we are confronted with instances of the instrumental use and abuse of shaming by those who have power in a church community. And yet there is no bitterness or cynicism in the book, quite the opposite: a strong emphasis on exploring what a healthy pastoral response looks like and what sort of Christian community it is that can be Christ-like in its handling of issues of shame. Nash does not hesitate to pass on many specific suggestions, actions, liturgical texts and practices from which any pastor is likely to find something they can readily use.

The book has two parts, 'Defining shame' and 'Confronting shame', and Nash helpfully structures her definition around six 'domains' of shame: personal, communal, relational, structural, theological, and historical. A note of caution: while the book is clearly structured and signposted, the main themes about experiences of shaming and exclusion in the church circle round and to some extent repeat through the chapters; however, this is no bad thing because in this way a momentum of awareness and indeed of indignation builds through the book. The author tells us that the chapters can be read to some extent independently of each other, and this is true: the book does not so much build an intellectual argument from front to back, as take us round many aspects of its main recurring themes.

There is concise, constructive material on biblical themes of shame, focussing mainly on classic narratives such as the fall, the woman caught in adultery, David, the woman with the haemorrhage, the prodigal son, although only the most passing reference is made to the significance of the cross. The author, wisely perhaps, does not spend much time on distinguishing between guilt and shame, noting Neil Pembroke's pithy formulation that 'guilt is about discrete actions, whereas shame encompasses the whole self' (170). However, sufficient consideration is given to the breadth of the concept of shame – drawing mainly on sources in psychology and social anthropology, as well as the important interdisciplinary work of Stephen Pattison and others; Nash gracefully acknowledges her personal debt to Pattison and to David Hewlett.

In welcoming this book, with its tight though apposite focus, one could mention other aspects of shame and shaming which might merit exploration by ethicists: firstly, Nash briefly alludes to the link between shame and rage (164), but there is a large theme here which could also be opened up – see, for example, James Gilligan on the roots of violence in shame. Also relevant here is the constructive use of shaming, in Maori culture in particular, which formed the cradle of the restorative justice movement (especially in the work of John Braithwaite on 'reintegrative shaming').

Secondly, the spiritual phenomenology of shame in terms of the human face encountering the face of God. The garden of Eden and the cross of Christ are mentioned in the book, but briefly. One might mention 'The Face of God' by the late and perhaps under-rated Catholic thinker Roger Scruton, and also reach back to Martin Buber and the personalist philosophy which flourished, especially in France, in the mid-20th century.

Thirdly, the prominence of the concept of shame in our discourse in the present century shows it is by no means only an ecclesiastical phenomenon. Shaming has become a major currency and a major

Crucible October 2021

concern in relation to many forms of discourse, especially social media, standing in fascinating interdependence with the correlative tendency to label others easily as being wonderful.

The blurb on the back of this book seems to suggest that all shame is bad. Sally Nash has a far more nuanced understanding than that. Her focus is unapologetically on the church, especially the local church, as her title makes clear. Walk through this book and, as a Crucible reader, you are likely to wince with recognition many times over, but also to find solid, practical resources for understanding experiences of shame and exclusion, and for countervailing pastoral practice.

Martin Kettle, Witney

Christianity Rediscovered: An Epistle from the Masai
Vincent J Donovan. Foreword by
Chris Lane.
SCM Press, 2019, 191pp, pbk, £12.99

Donovan's classic first appeared in 1978 and, rather remarkably, his main thesis remains as challenging as ever, written with simplicity and appeal. Having in the intervening years visited Tanzania a number of times, including the Masai country, the picture felt to this reviewer still more vivid. Of course, geopolitics have changed but the essential message is unaffected. Quoting an American university student in relation to that message, Donovan writes: 'You must have the courage to go with them to a place that neither you nor they have ever been before' (xiv).

The missionary history of the region is traced in broad outline, including the influence of the Arab traders early on, the subsequent buying of slaves' freedom and then the 'quid pro quo' of enforced conversion. The shift to a proper focus on health and education follows with the work of Catholic mission orders, including the part played by Father Arthur (later Cardinal) Hinsley. The credit side of all this is noted (especially the humanitarian impact) but the debit side too; the institutionalisation of mission and evangelism with the deadweight of buildings, little focus on liturgy and virtually no indigenisation even in terms of clergy. Often there was little mention of religion or talk of God.

The glamour and attractiveness of the Masai is well captured, as is the contrasting cultural background, utterly different from western ways. For example, there is no future tense in the Masai language – so resurrection becomes a double mystery! Donovan, in his 'letter to the bishop', as he prepares for mission in Tanzania outlines a very different approach, both 'travelling light' in terms of buildings, and sitting light to conventional ways of framing the Gospel. He calls as witnesses to his approach writers who had been long forgotten, including the Anglican, Roland Allen. Allen's writings went back as far as 1913. The approach to mission outlined in Vatican II and that implied in St Paul's letters are contrasted.

Exploring the Masais' perception of the 'High God', he then asked them 'what do you think of the Christ'? Listening to their responses, dramatically he writes: 'Man (humanity) is God appearing in the universe' (p.70) – this is Incarnation, and a contemporary take on Christian humanism. Moving to the Church and Baptism, the full challenge of western individualism makes its impact. Descartes is foresworn and his dictum rephrased for the life of the human community. So, how can the Masai describe what we know as the Church? Ultimately the nearest that Donovan can come to translating this is 'the age-group brother of God'. Masai civilisation can be seen only in community terms and this, of course, has clear lessons for western culture. Such issues are still sharper now as the digital age has taken us further into our own virtual shells.

Next we are offered a charming introduction to Ole Sikii, a young Masai with an extraordinary religious sensibility, a born liturgist in terms of his own indigenous religion. He even walked seventy-five miles to climb a volcano and seek out the remote high God in whom he believed. Later we read of him fighting a leopard which had terrified his village and killing it with nothing but his own bare hands. Ole becomes one of the most effective catechists with his own people, telling them of baptism and of the Christian faith.

For all his revolutionary methods, there is no overestimating the conviction with which Donovan conveyed the Gospel. The key is to proclaim it and then leave allowing the community to develop their faith, but without the western and European assumptions about what the Church is and of what it must be comprised. Priesthood must be re-imagined and the Gospel seen to be no part of any system, Marxist, Capitalist or whatever.

The final chapter, titled 'The Winds of Change', plays on words used by Harold Macmillan in his famous speech to the South African

Parliament in 1960, when he spoke of 'a wind of change' blowing throughout Africa. From there, Donovan concludes with a carefully restated definition of missionary work which he then analyses phrase by phrase. 'The recapitulation of all things in Christ is what is in store for the human race', he notes (p.181). Keriko , a Masai catechist, tells the gospel story in memorable phrases from his own culture – it is beautiful, moving and a succinct capturing of the faith. The brief African Creed concluding the book is a summary of the message. Forty two years on, this book remains unique – if you have not read it, then here is the chance. Having read it many years ago, I was more than refreshed by its energy and faith.

Stephen Platten, Berwick-upon-Tweed

The Hebrew Bible and Environmental Ethics: Humans, Nonhumans, and the Living Landscape
Mari Joerstad
Cambridge University Press, 2019, 246pp, hbk, £75

The Cry of the Earth and the Cry of the Poor: Hearing Justice in John's Gospel
Kathleen P Rushton
SCM Press, 2020, 256pp, pbk, £25

Mari Joerstad's exploration of environmental ethics in the Hebrew Bible is fascinating. Proceeding from the idea that poetic phrases like 'the earth devours', 'mountains skip', or 'trees clap their hands' are not merely metaphors, but expressions of belief that non-human, even non-animal, natural entities are worthy of respect, interaction, and of being recognized as in active relationship with God, Joerstad believes that they can, in fact, be regarded as 'persons'. This treads a careful line between animism, where nature is inhabited by spirits or deities, and the idea that non-human entities are merely objects: 'either gods or stage dressing', as Joerstad puts it. The natural world, created before humanity, has a value to God in its own right, obeying God's will and co-operating with God in upholding justice.

Non-human persons have God-given roles and responsibilities. Astronomical bodies distinguish day and night and order time; the earth produces plants; animals spread out and multiply; landscape

61

features 'witness' not only God's acts of creation, but human behaviour, decisions and vows. Similarly to feminist understandings of Biblical taboos about women revealing them to be more compassionate than punitive, taking the perspective of the objects of Hebrew dietary laws brings those laws into focus as more about species protection, than as value-judgements on 'clean' or 'unclean' animals.

Joerstadt's approach makes sense of two perennially puzzling books. Instead of pussy-footing around the Song of Songs as an allegory of love between God and humanity, she sees the blending of nature settings and imagery – 'lovers-as-gardens, lovers-in-gardens' – as a unification of human and natural life, ruptured by disobedience in Genesis, but now restored by love. The Book of Job's glorious descriptions of nature seem more of a non-sequitur than an answer, in the face of Job's suffering; but just as climate scientists tell us that Earth will endure, even if humans die out, Job's problems assume different proportions when he realizes that 'outside of Job's attention is a whole world that does not care about Job.'

This, Joerstad admits, is not cosy, with no room for us humans to feel special – and she admits that the scriptures are capable of more than one interpretation. She concludes by analysing various ethical approaches in the context of this world view, and finds more sympathy in artistic responses – including landscape gardening – which show co-operation with nature and reflect our nurturing by it. Her final chapter, 'Befriending the World', ends with the hope we will discover anew that it is a companiable and hospitable place.

Kathleen Rushton explains that 'connection with eco- and biosphere, expressing the interconnected relationship with God, the land and the people' – very much Joerstad's thesis – '[was] Jesus' inherited tradition'. Modelled on the 'lectio divina' cycle, she accompanies her commentaries on the Sunday lections from St John's Gospel with hints on mindful reading, suggestions for prayer, action points for hearing and responding to 'the cry of the earth and the cry of the poor' – and incidentally provides much useful fuel for sermon-preparation.

Rushton's approach to eco-theology is conventional, but uncovering environmental messages in John often requires some imagination. She encourages meditations on water, walking, pilgrimage, celebration. The gathering of leftovers after feeding the five thousand reminds us to care for places and avoid waste. Neil Armstrong's awe at seeing Earth from space and appreciating its fragility is cited with no sense of irony at the environmental cost of the space programme.

Crucible October 2021

There is, as Rushton points out, plenty of bucolic imagery in John: harvests, wheat, barley, wine, water, shepherding, village weddings, convivial meals – but are they always what they seem? Barley loaves shared with the five thousand are the hard-won food of the poor, calling to mind the dependence of the whole community on sweated labour, contrasting their abundance with the all-too-common experience of scarcity. Village weddings uphold traditional male-female divisions, a wine-shortage risks dishonouring the family, and it's OK for a son to speak patronisingly to his mother. But in light of 'The Lord is my shepherd,' is it fair to say that 'good shepherds' were virtually unheard-of in Israel, and the 'noble shepherd' draws more from Greek than Hebrew literature? And are the many points where Jesus is identified with Wisdom/Sophia – from presence at creation to inviting us to share bread and wine – entirely positive, or do they incline towards supplanting the divine feminine with a male character?

Rushton's commentaries reveal intriguing details. Nicodemus – pillar of the Jewish establishment, visiting Jesus by night, not quite believing – contrasts with the Samaritan woman who meets Jesus in the blazing light of noon, grasps the point of 'living water', and becomes an evangelist for the Good News. The Eastern Church names her Photini, and although she personifies the heavy, time-consuming labour that remains a daily chore for millions of women, Rushton invites us to see Photini's mid-day trip to the well as not so much a sign of her unpopularity, as illustrative of 'walking in the light' she recognizes in Jesus. Hard-working Martha, meanwhile, 'ministers' to the company instead of acting as domestic servant: a neat reversal of the usual associations of using the same word as for 'Deacon' in the early church.

Fascinatingly, both authors tell similar stories of modern, urban people struggling to comprehend indigenous societies' identification with place. Joerstad mentions an American researcher utterly unable to follow the conversation of his Apache friends, when their exchange consisted entirely of place-names; Rushton describes a conference-leader inviting participants to introduce themselves with the traditional Maori reference to 'my mountain' and 'my river'. Do try it: like these examples, both books open up new and challenging ways of seeing ourselves, our scriptures and the world around us.

Carol Wardman, Ceredigion

Crucible October 2021

Does Religion do More Harm than Good?
Rupert Shortt
SPCK, 2019, 80pp, pbk, £9.99

Religion Hurts: Why religions do harm as well as good
John Bowker
SPCK, 2018, 176pp, hbk, £14.99

Neither of these books are for the faint hearted in search of easy answers. The intellectual quality of both texts demonstrate that it is possible to capture, crystalise and communicate complexity with care and an even-handed judgement. For those so immersed in the flow of the water of religion we might do well to stand back and think about the nature of religion and its paradoxes.

Shortt addresses his organising question with energy and fluency – what are we to make of religion? How should we evaluate the claims and counter claims of the effects of religion on society? Arguments are assessed and judgements made. We are reminded that the negativity and cynicism about religion are popular in 'our age of growing endarkenment'. The nature of truth, the relationship of religion and politics and debates between science and theology all serve to question the rationality and efficacy of religious truth and practice.

These areas are mined with thoughtful reflexivity. The power of secularism and its distortions are faced, and the book balances them with a clear articulation that religion does indeed do more good than harm. Love and happiness can never be controlled, captured or packaged. Heartful mystery lies at the centre of the striving for flourishing. Religion can help us mature, to know ourselves as bounded and to bid us into a richer and generative change where dependence and freedom balance complex ambiguities.

While 'maturity' is attractive for all who seek meaning, Shortt helpfully makes a distinction between good and bad religion. The dangers and consequences of intolerance are named especially when this leads to violence but balanced by the empowerment of believers to love especially the vulnerable and stranger in their midst. This has been evidenced by the responses of many faith traditions in the Covid pandemic in their localities and neighbourhoods.

This book deserves to be read both by those who want to rethink their views of religion but also by some who are embedded in institutional religious life which may lead to a complacency that lacks wisdom. His reader is bidden (and enabled) to think - and think more deeply.

Bowker deals with similar territory. How are we to understand the nature of religion and its often-complex variety of convictions and practices? Where are we to find the balance between the power of the good in religion and its obvious destructive toxicities? Bowker brings his decades of scholarship to bear upon these questions and the claims of religion as it shapes our evolution and development as human beings.

The skill of this text is the quality of both its connectivity and synergies. Ethics, philosophy, anthropology, history are put to work as the chapters hold the tensions between reason and emotion and the realities of the good and the evil present in all religions. This becomes especially acute when religion, for very good reasons attempts to exercise power in the social and political realms of public life. Self-interest, altruism and misguiding actions are all part of our global ecology where even the best of intentions can have hideous consequences. We might consider ongoing ethical debates about gender and sexual identity as examples of this. The way we construct (or defend) a world view through our religious metaphors and languages shapes and distorts our human flourishing.

Bowker also believes in the power of religion to shape the common good. He believes that we need to address many of the questions that Islam poses and indeed that Christian- Islamic engagement could be a route into great peace and understanding of the evolving realities of human society

Bowker invites his reader into the adventure of exploration and discovery, of looking at the pictures and stories that religion offers for us to understand our life and its paradoxes. These enable us to deal with matters of life and death, of meaning and creativity, of the place of myth and ritual in our endeavours. This leads Bowker to show us that religion in all its many textured colours needs to be taken more and not less seriously.

Two excellent books that offer a model of good writing. Less can be more and a wider interdisciplinary perspective (perhaps especially in the world of Christian ethics) might be able to bring us more focus and wisdom into the particularities of the present moment. This may well be a key task in these months ahead as we engage in our post-lockdown recovery. How can religion enable us to be theologically generative ?

James Woodward, Sarum College and the University of Winchester

HYMNS Ancient & Modern

Crucible

Please complete section 1. Cheque **or** 2. Credit/Debit card **or** 3. Direct debit
**(the name and address you give must match the information
on your credit/Debit card/bank statement.)**

YOUR DETAILS (Please complete]

Title ....Christian name ....Surname ....

Address: ....

....

....

Postcode .... Daytime telephone no ....

Email: ....

- I enclose a cheque for the total amount of £..............
  payable to Hymns Ancient and Modern Ltd.
- To pay by credit/debit card please visit www.cruciblejournal.co.uk/subscribe
  or contact us on 01603 785911

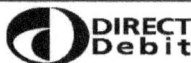

www.ingramcontent.com/pod-product-compliance
Lightning Source LLC
Chambersburg PA
CBHW032154020426
42334CB00016B/1279